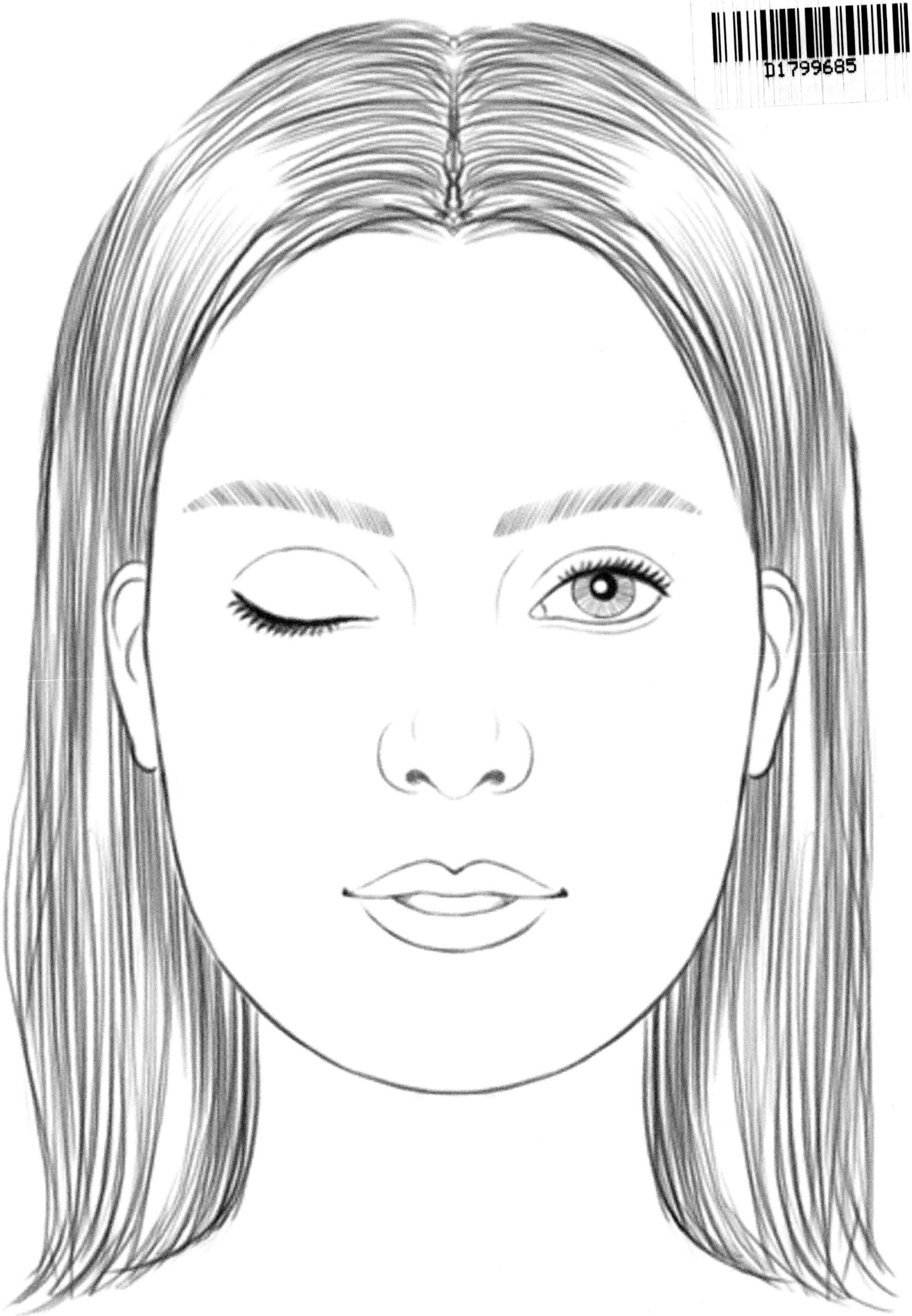

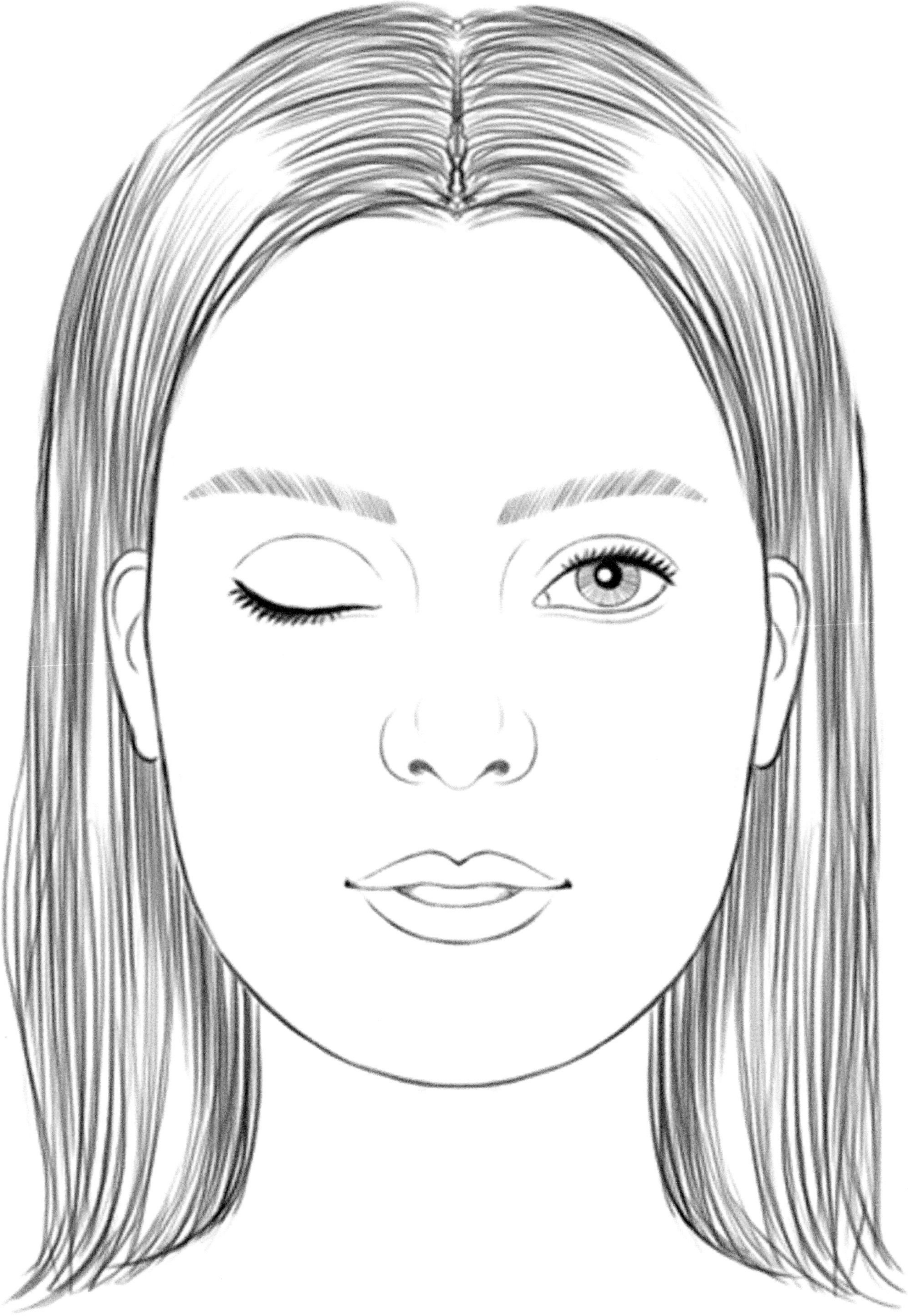

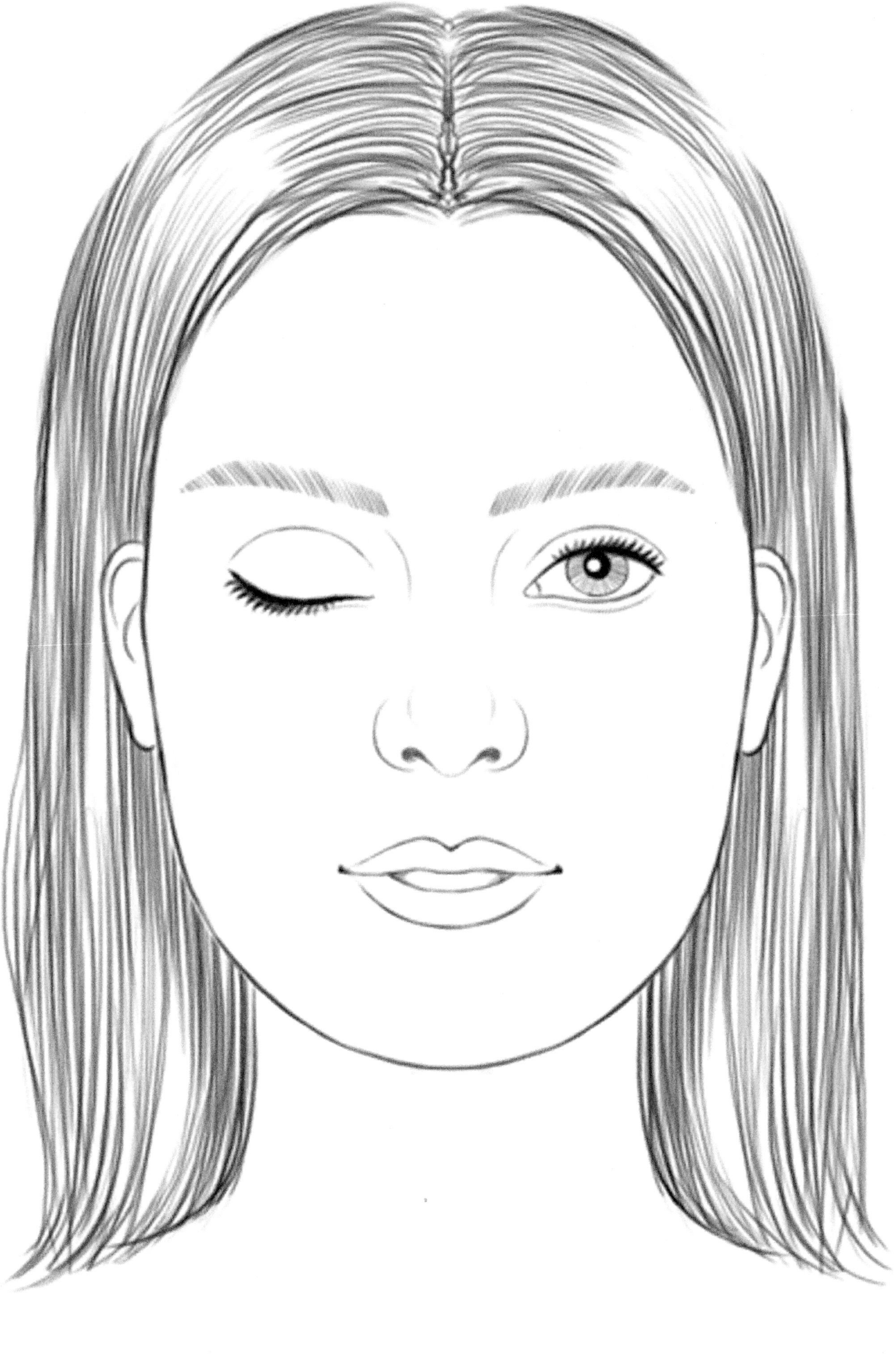

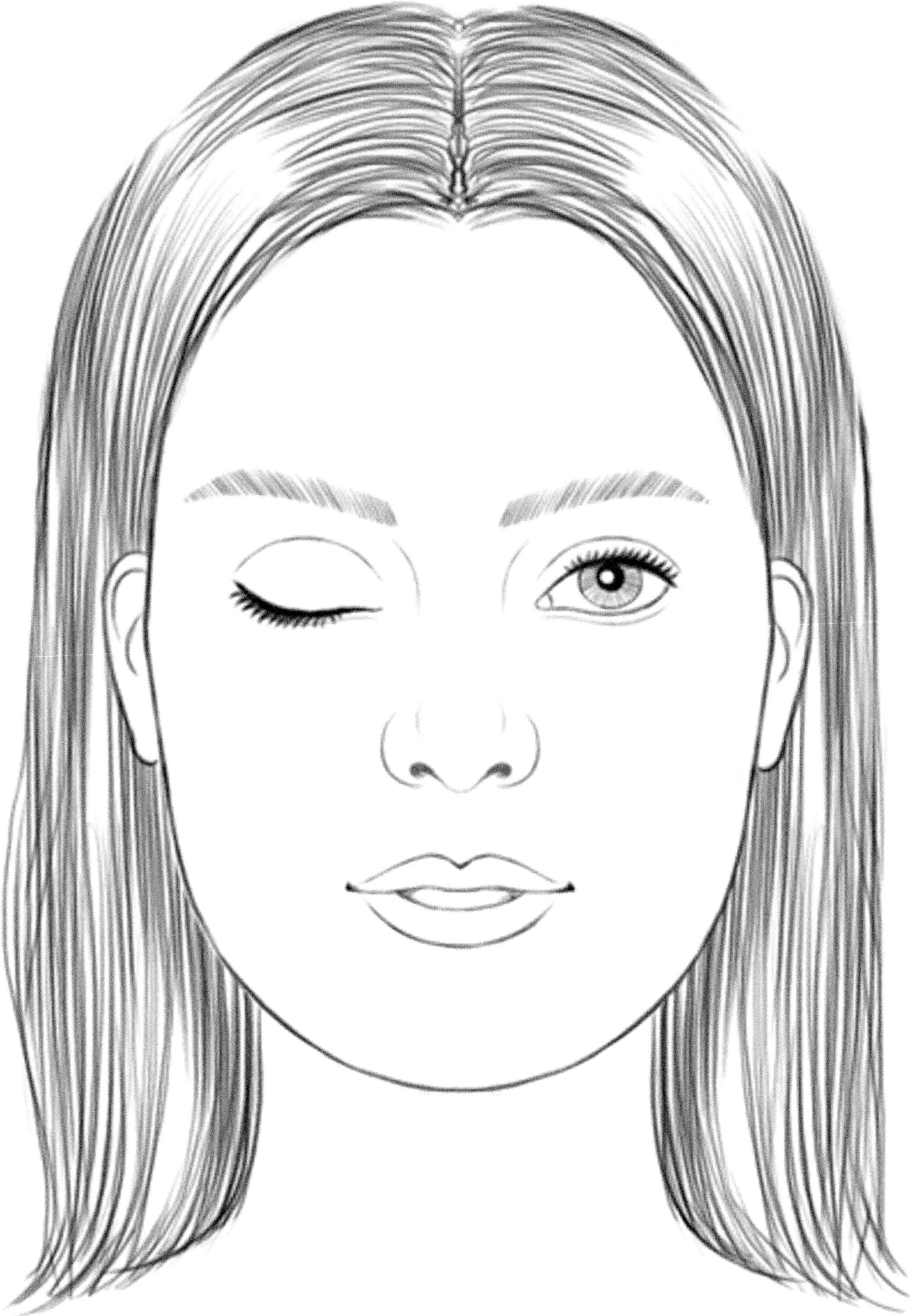

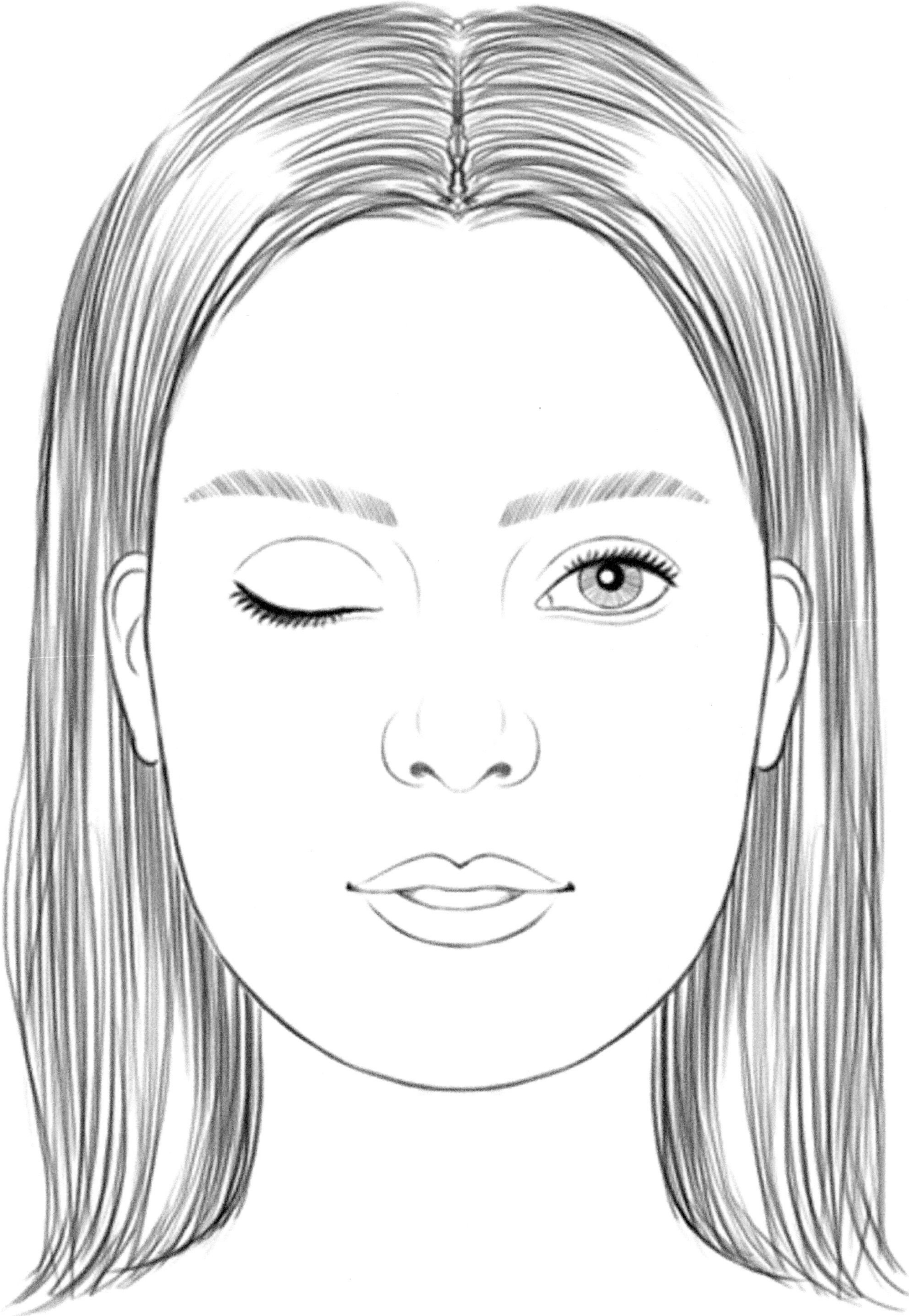

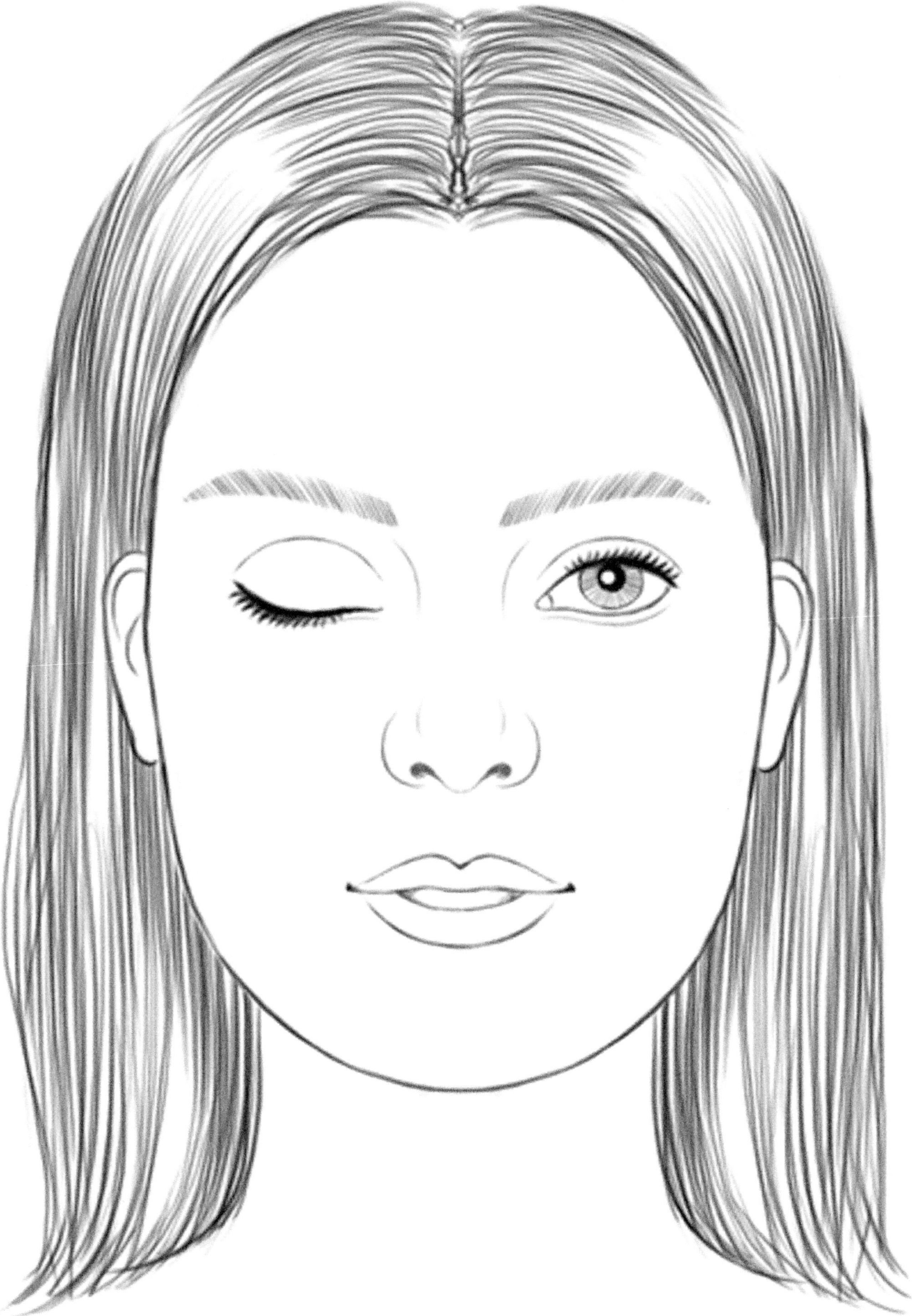

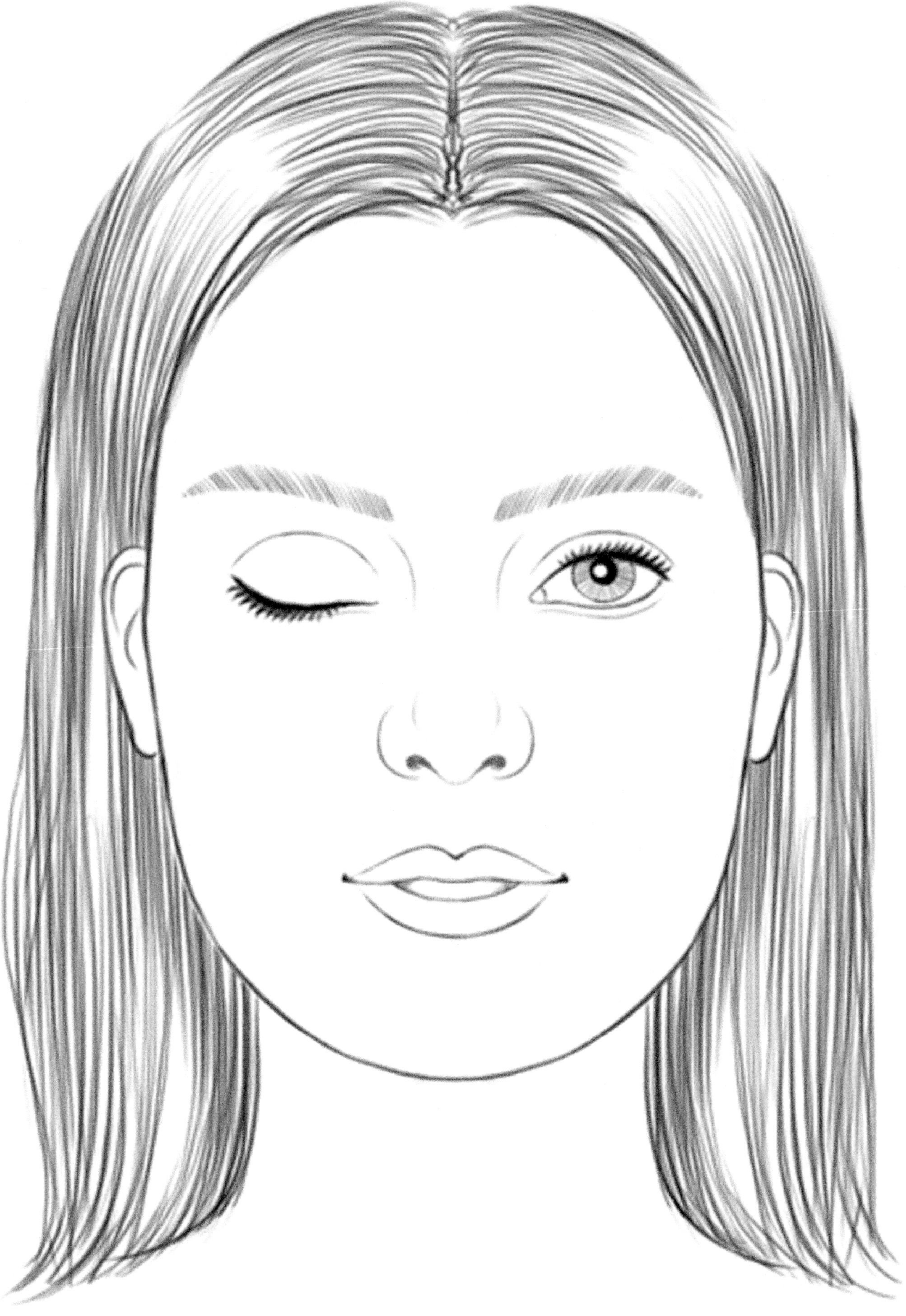

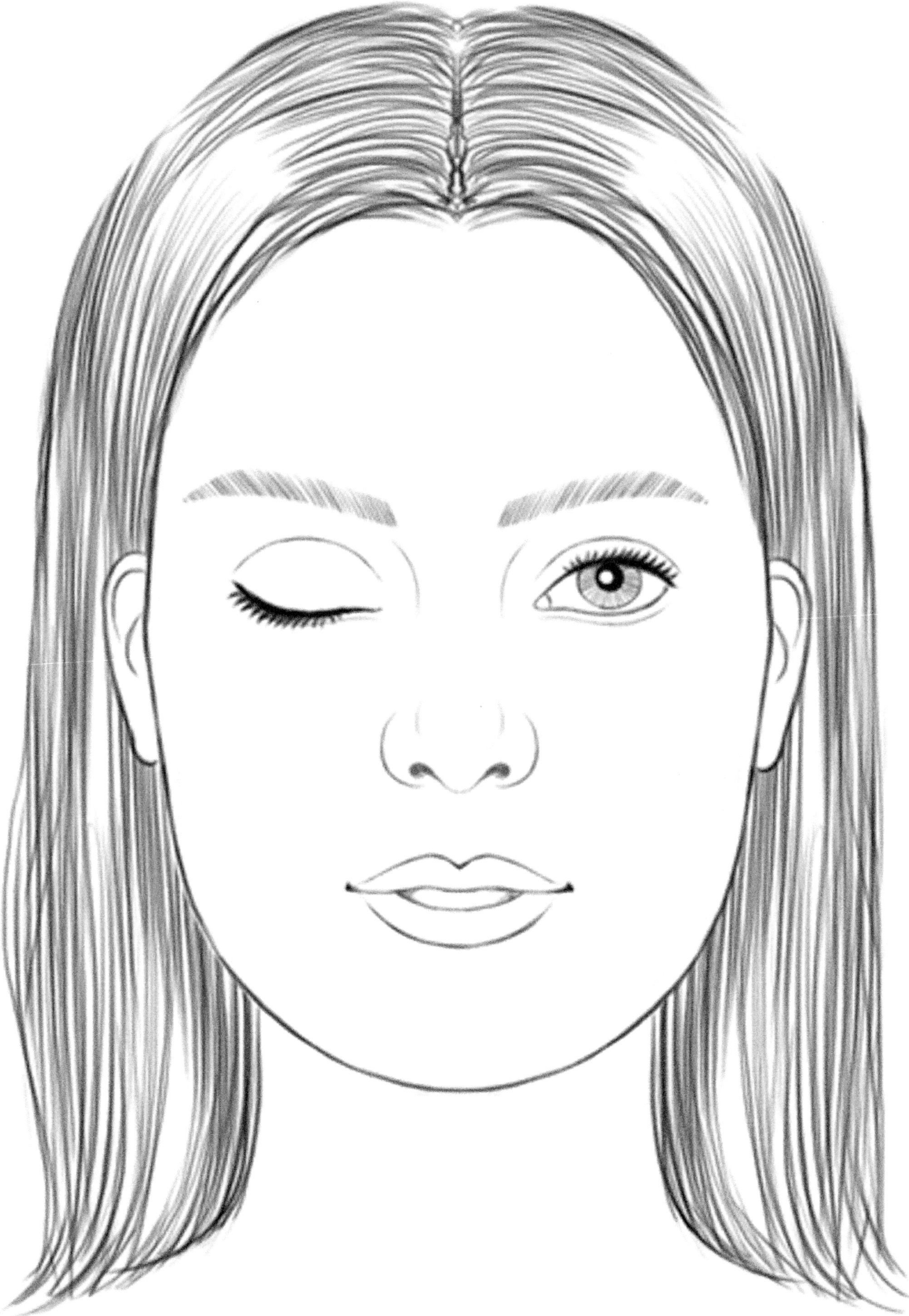

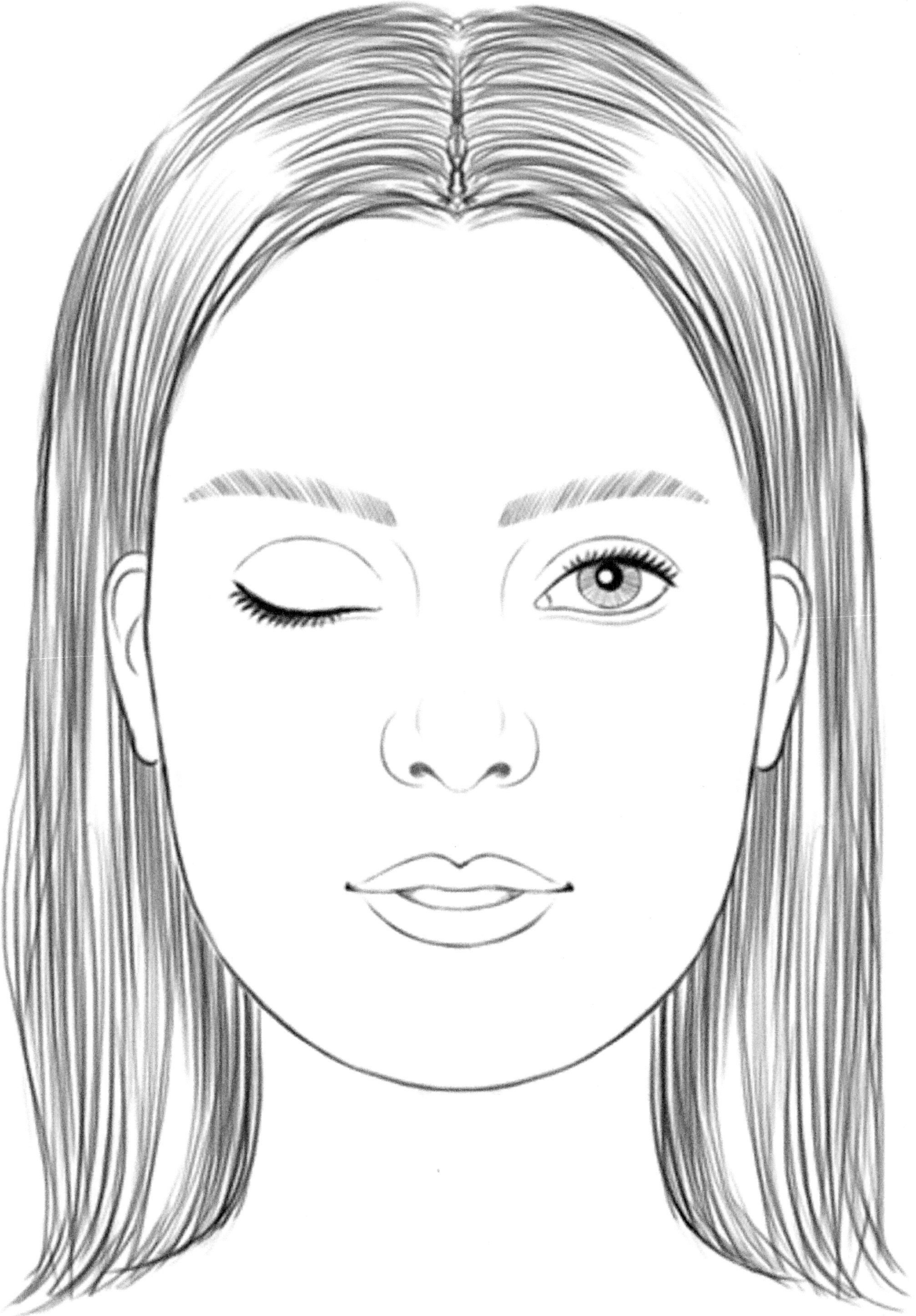

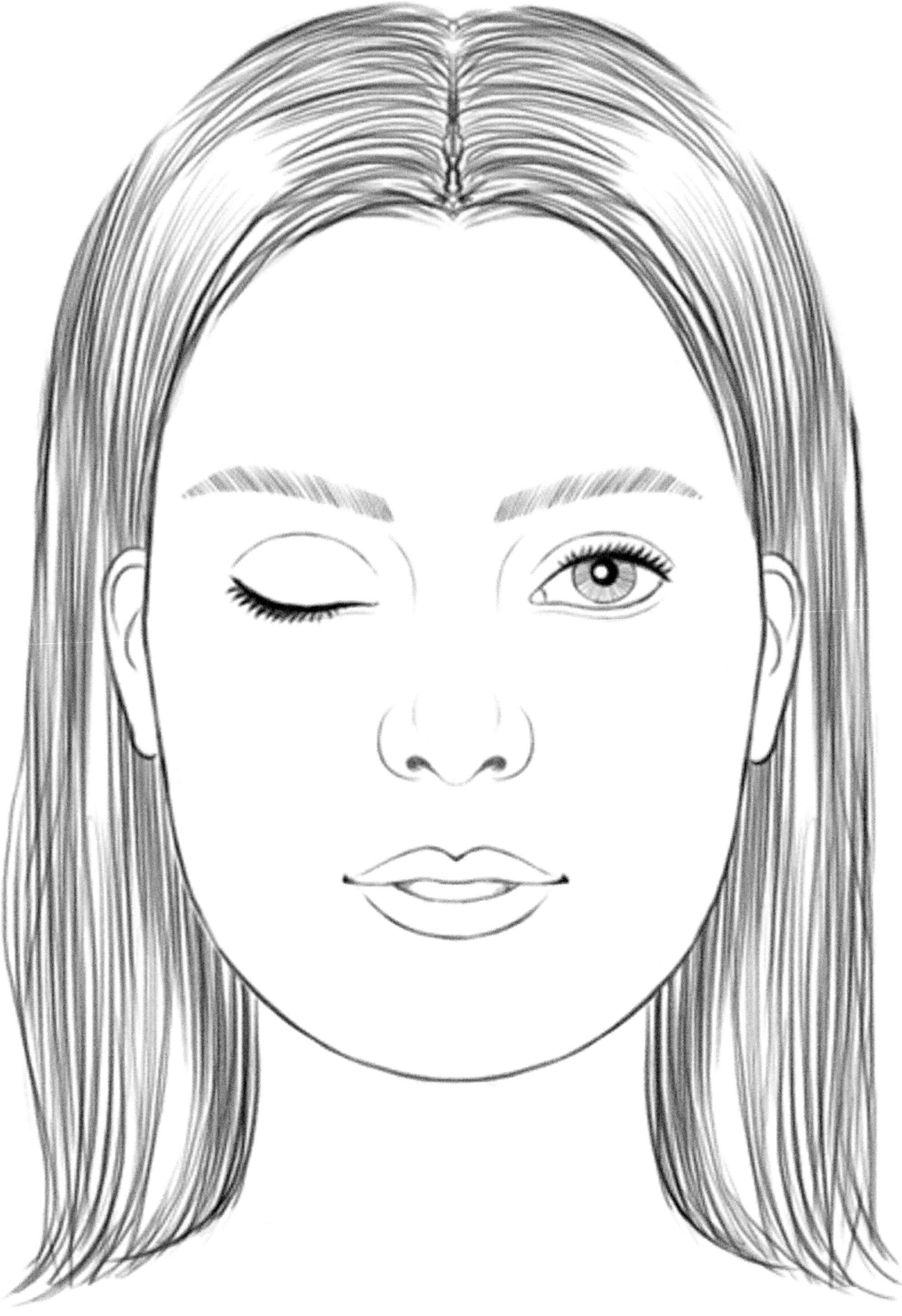

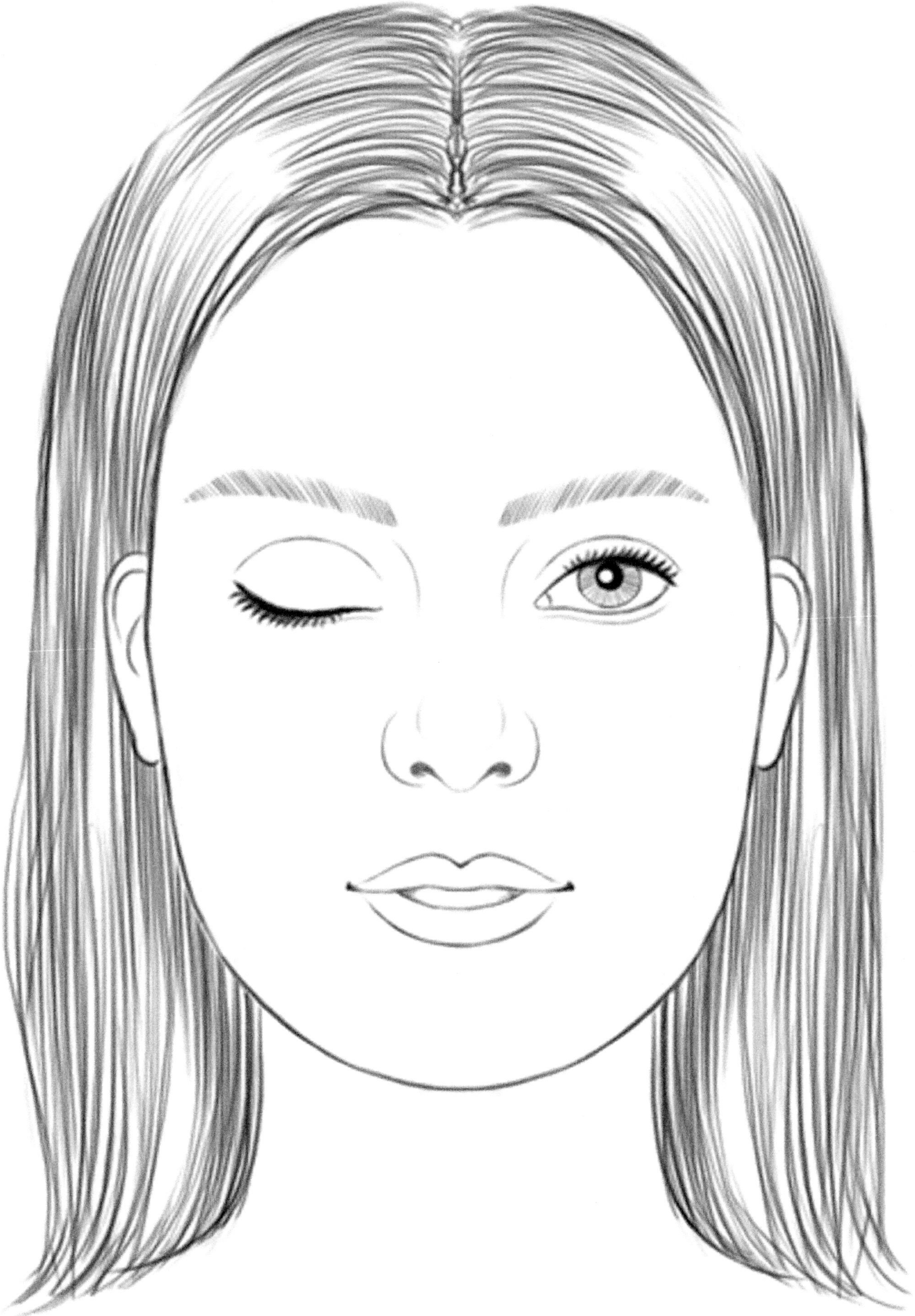

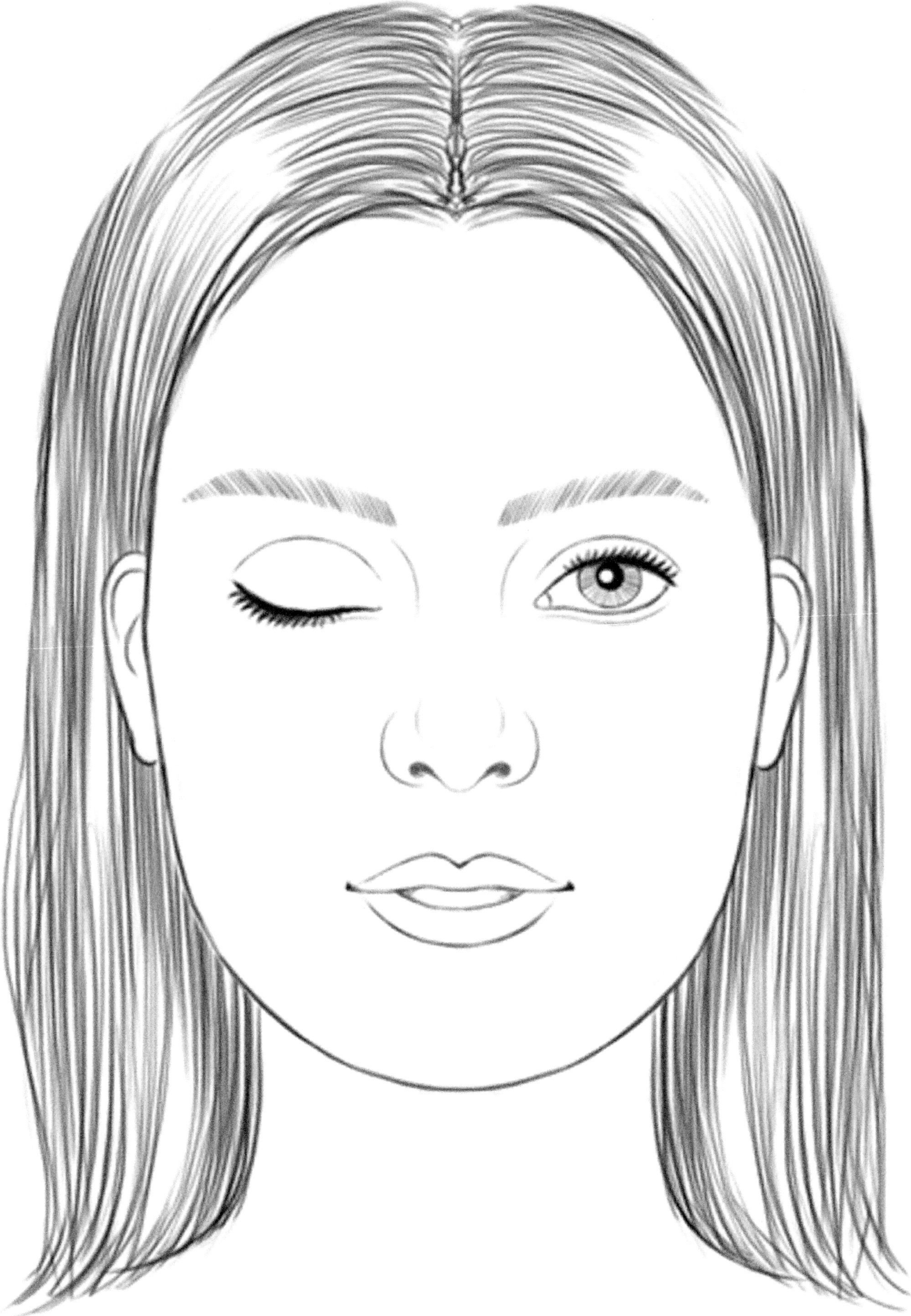

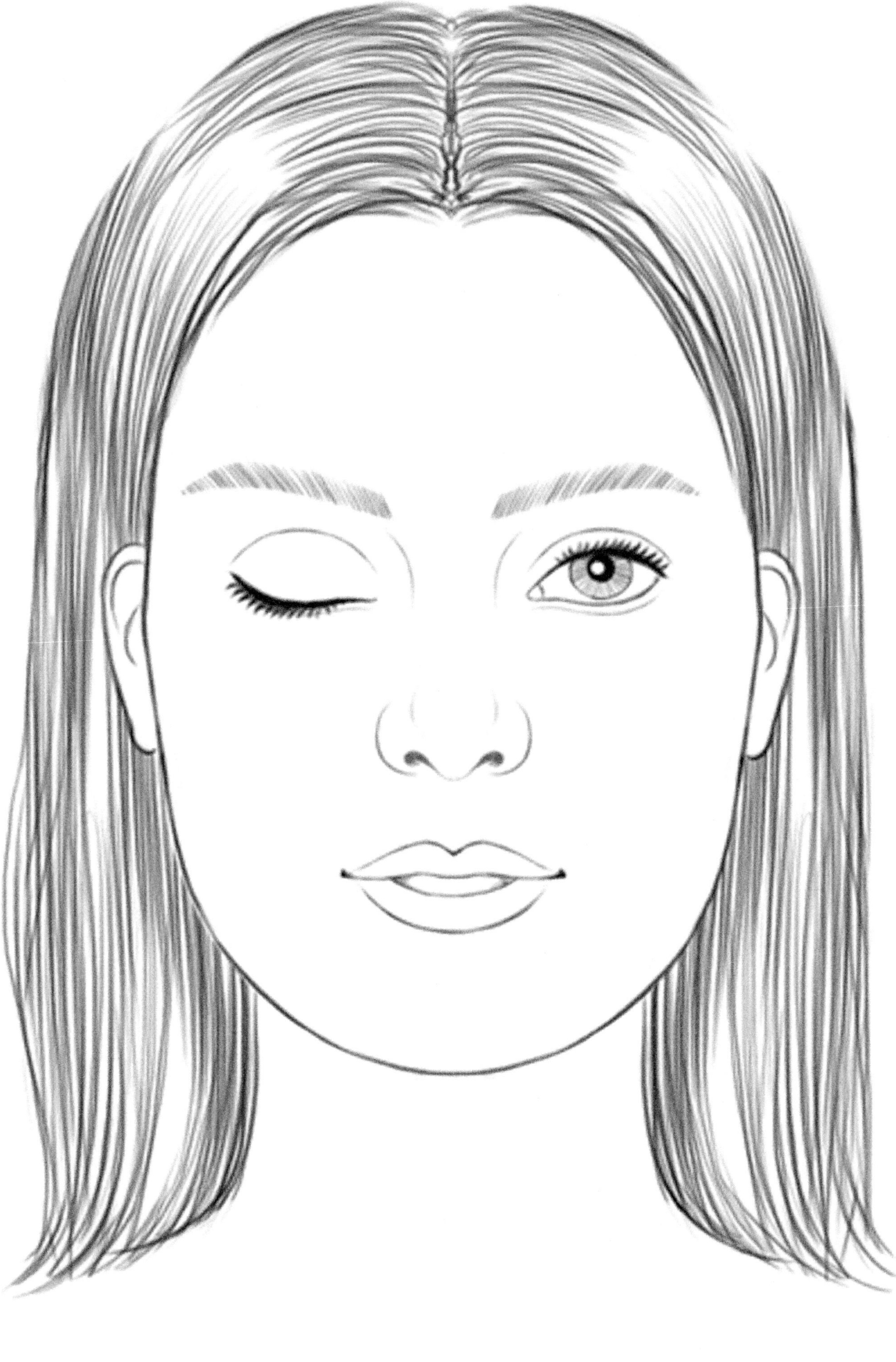

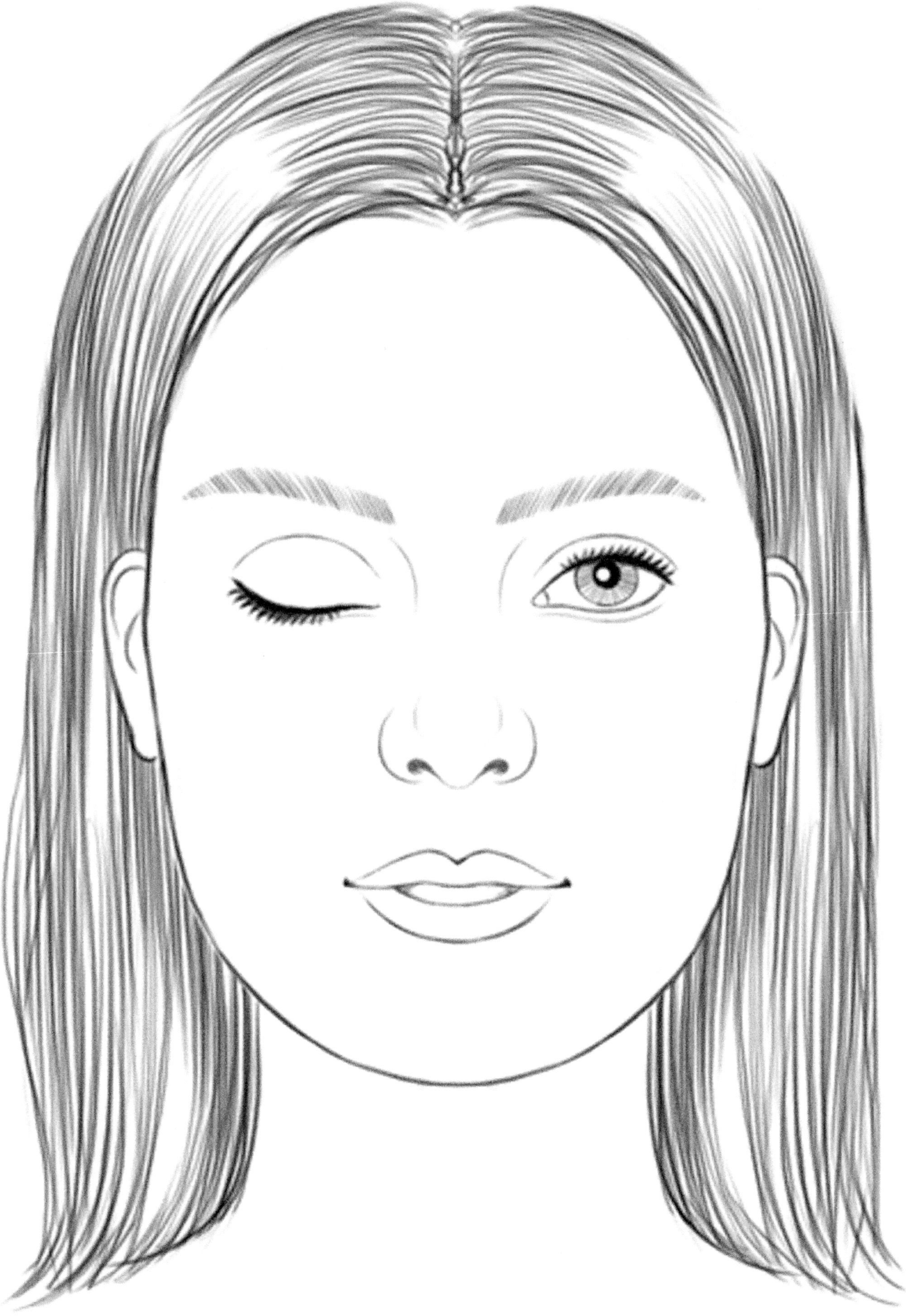

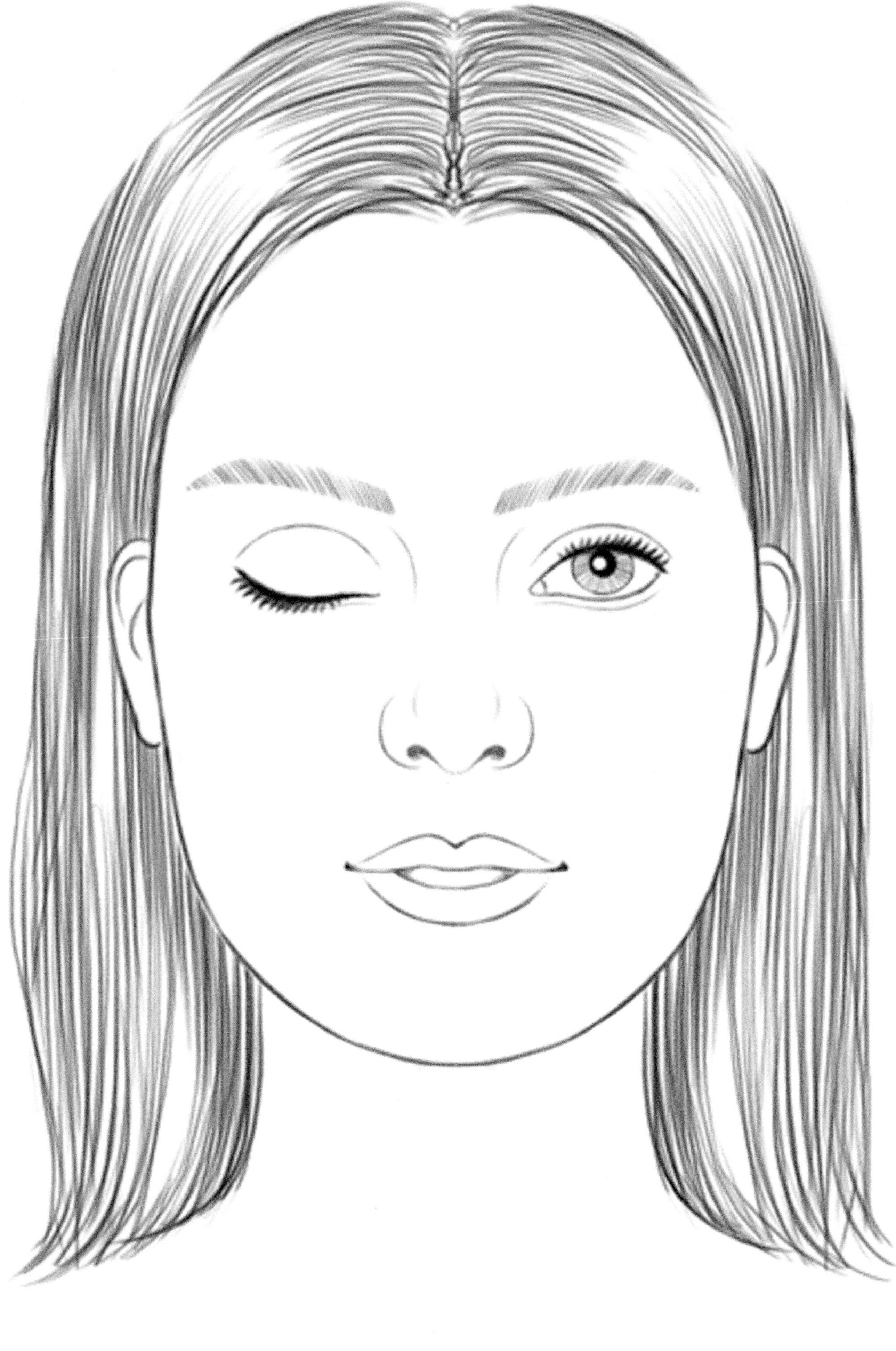

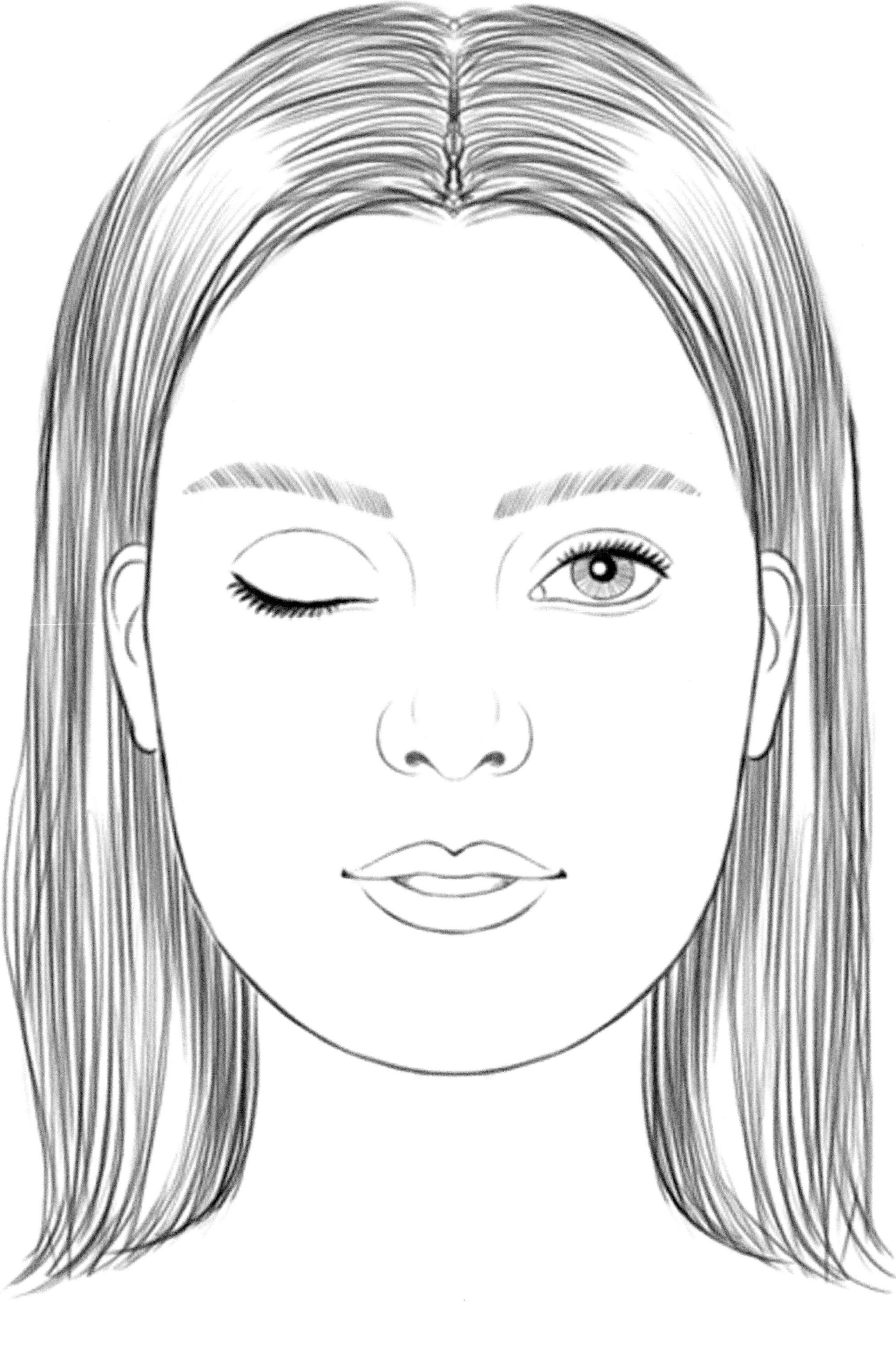

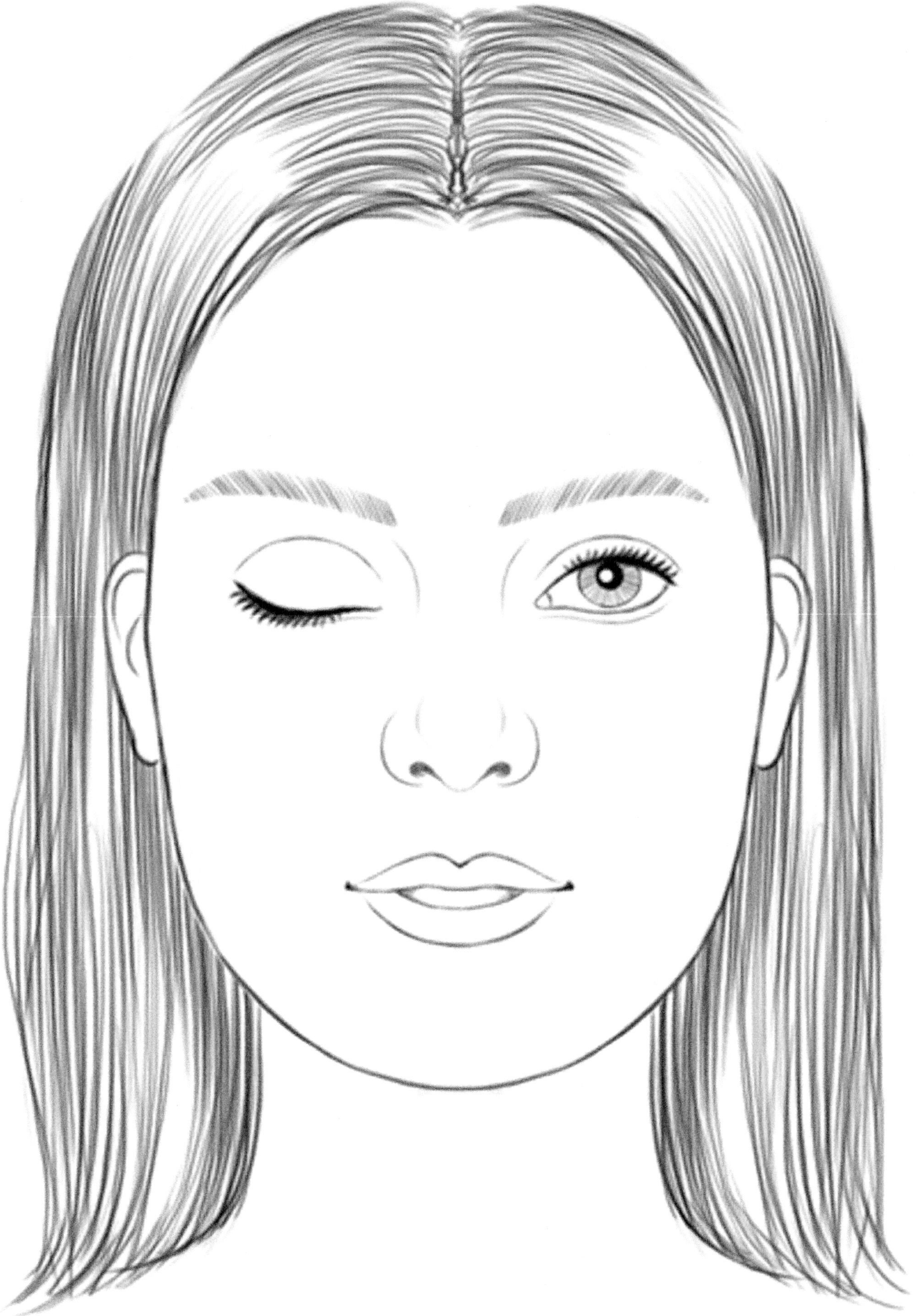

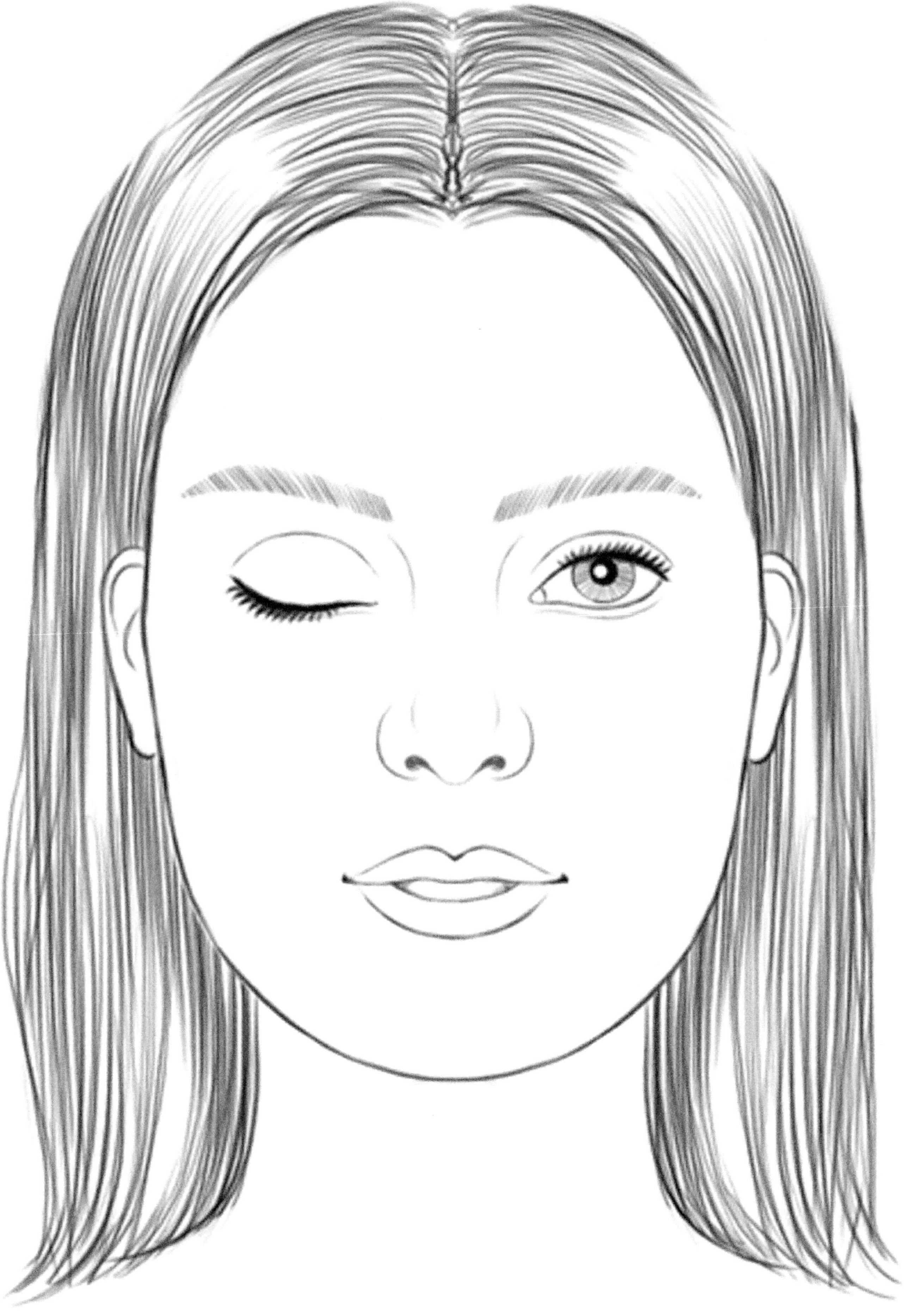

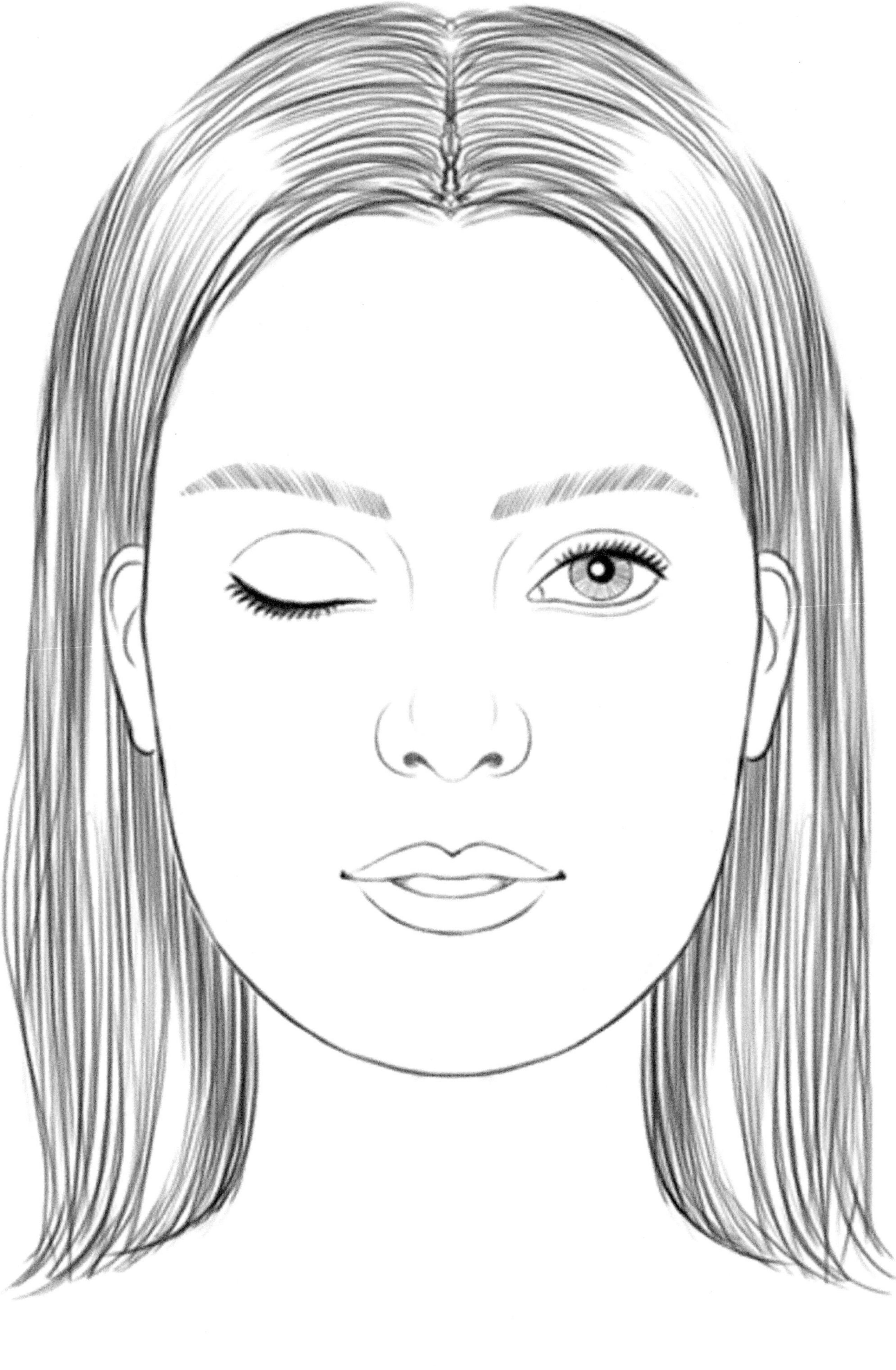

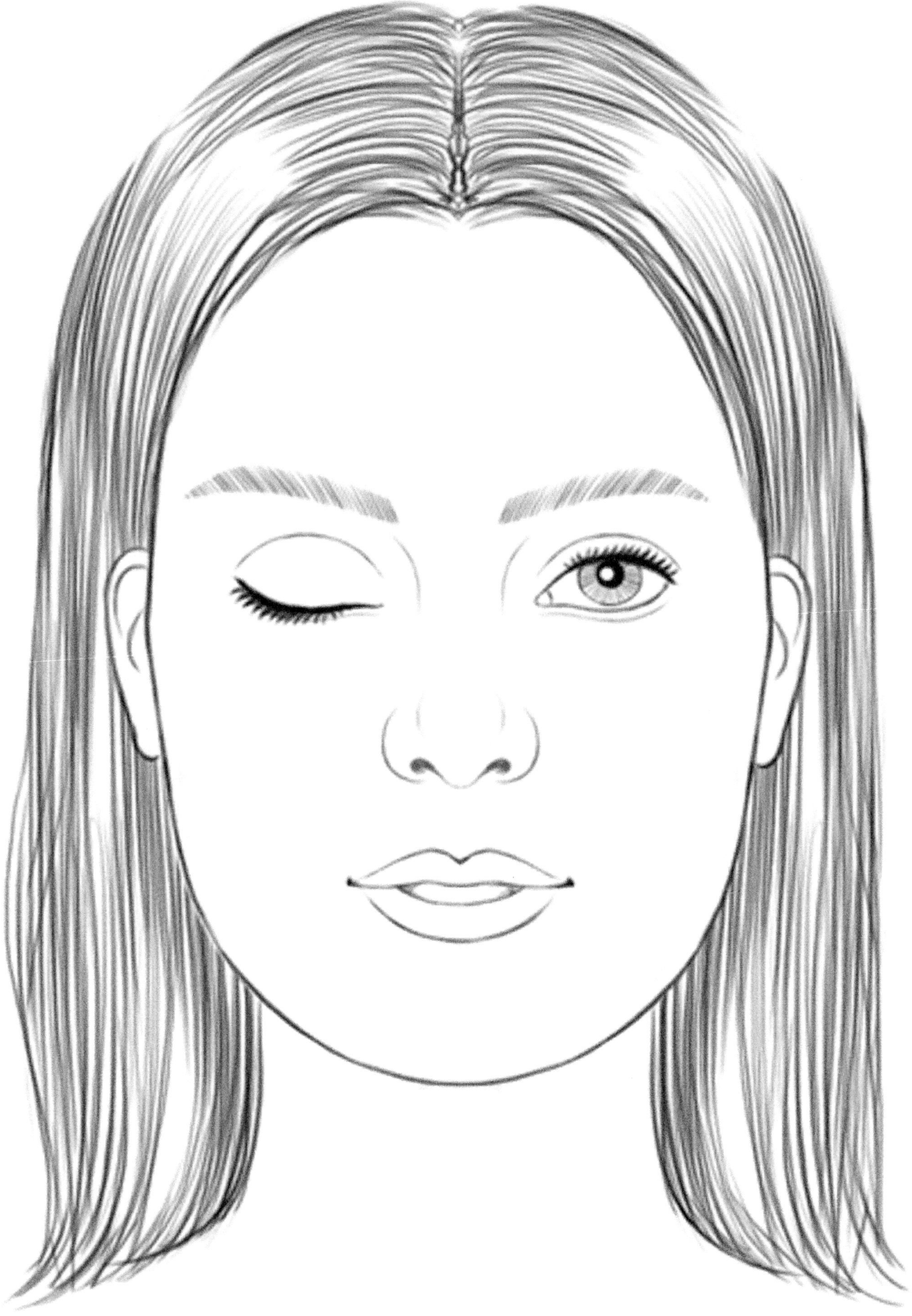

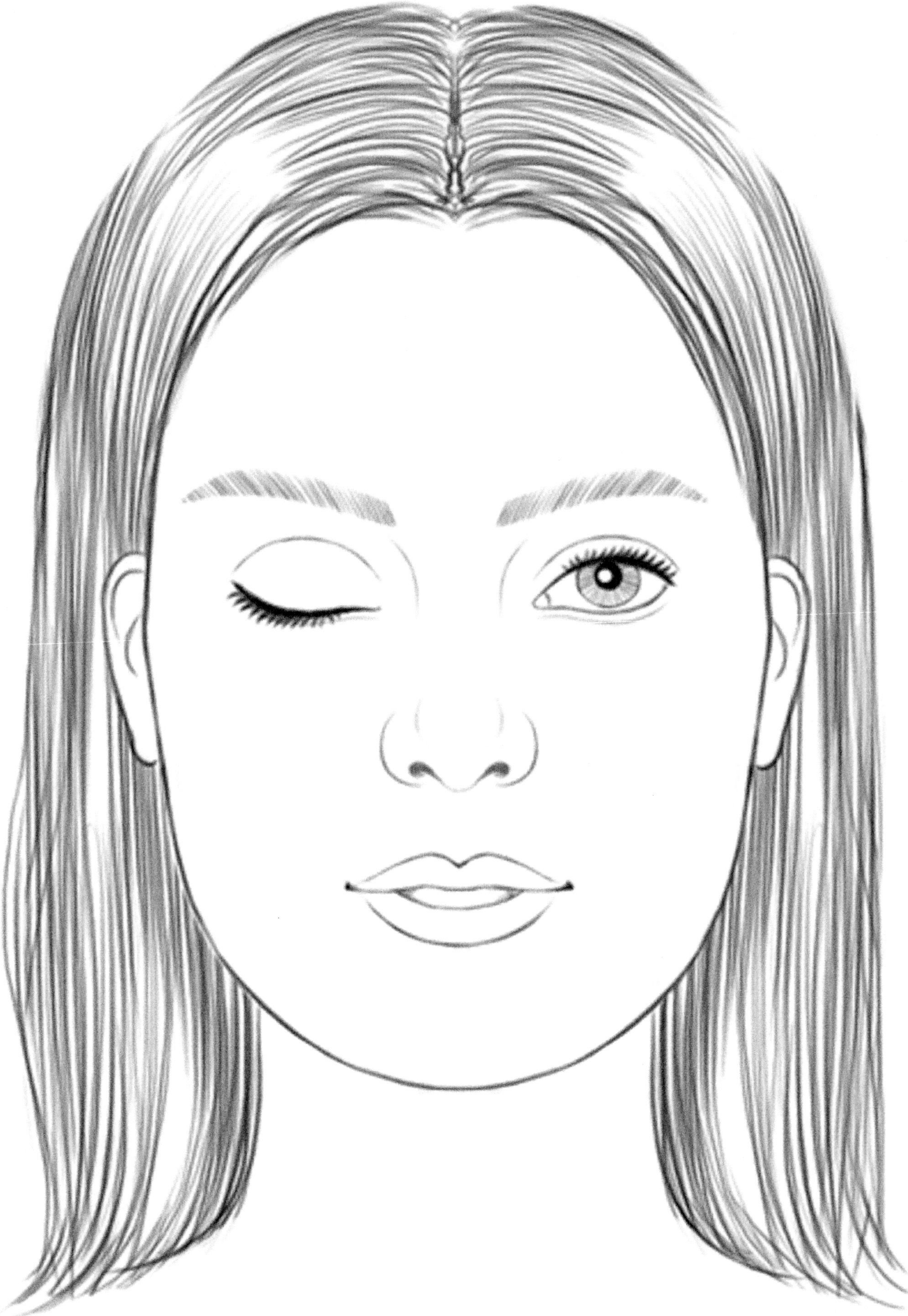

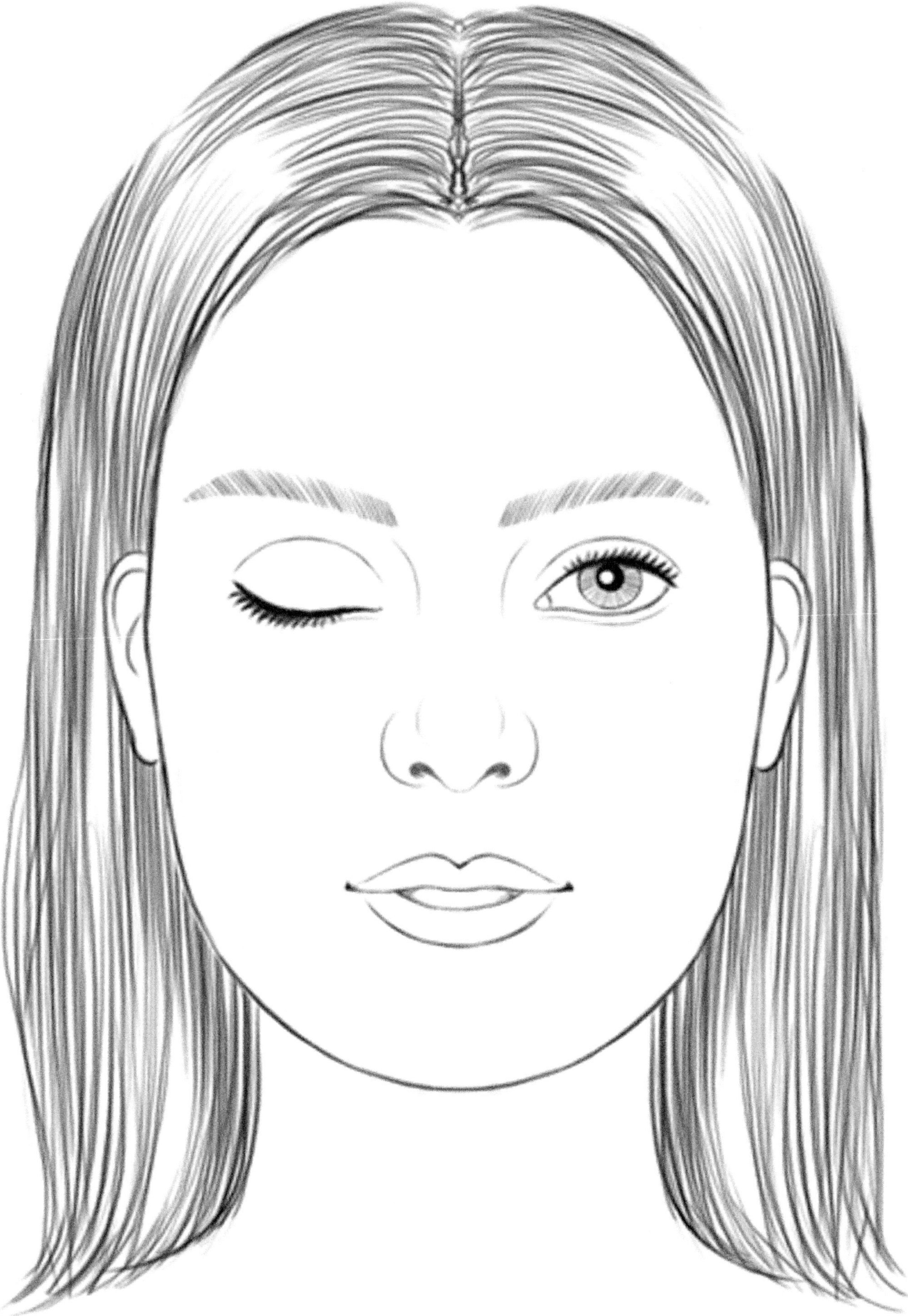

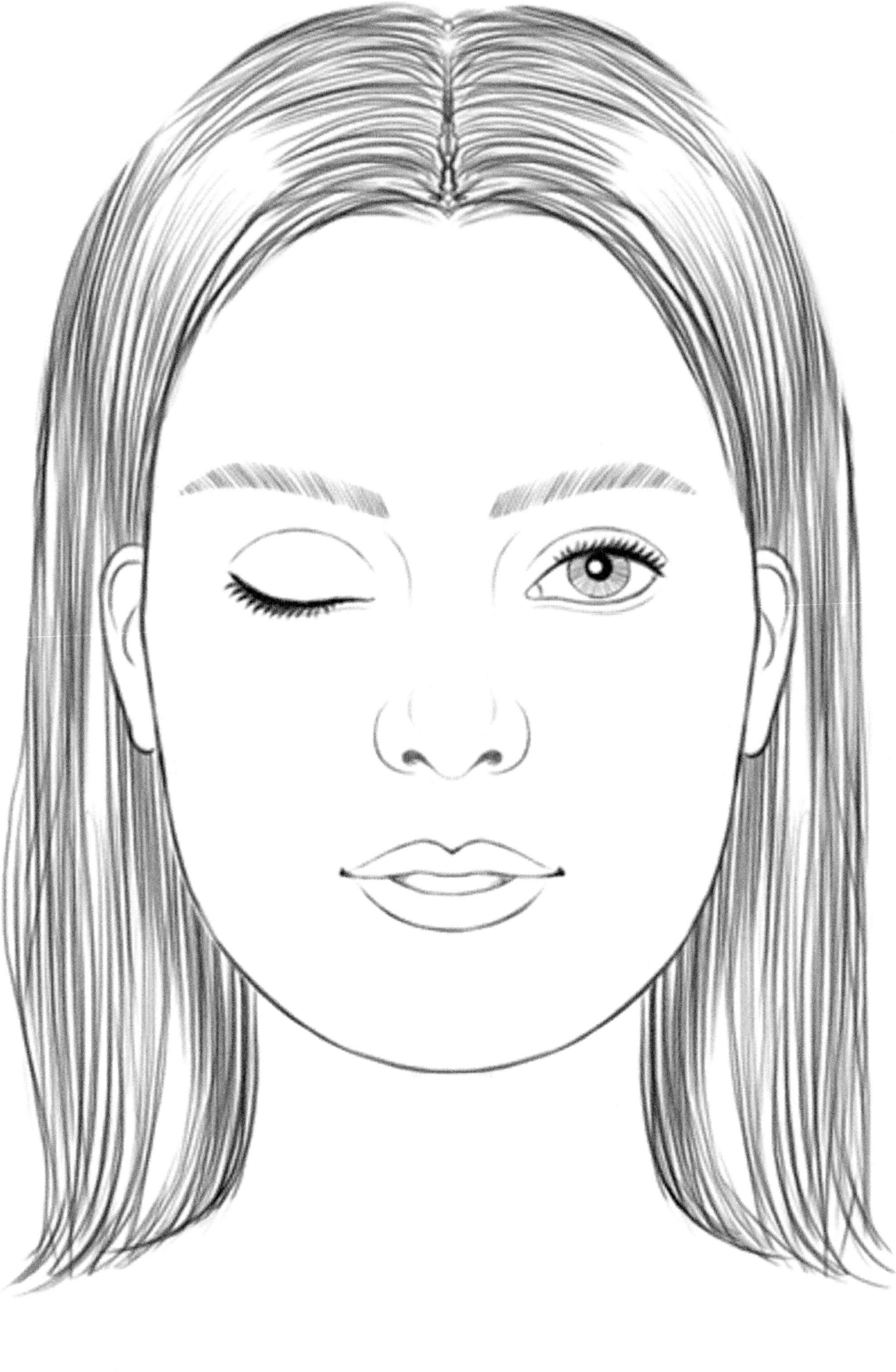

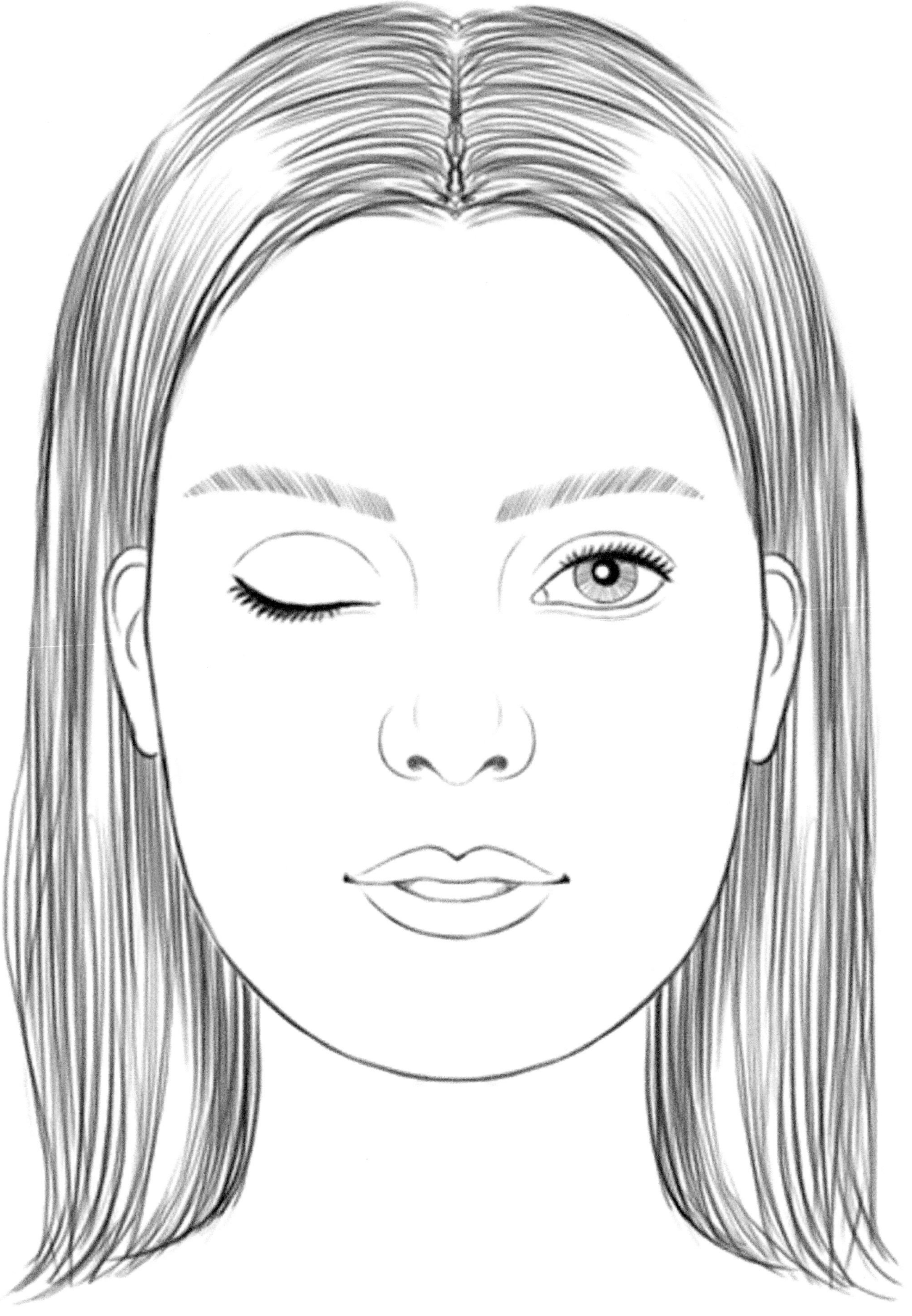

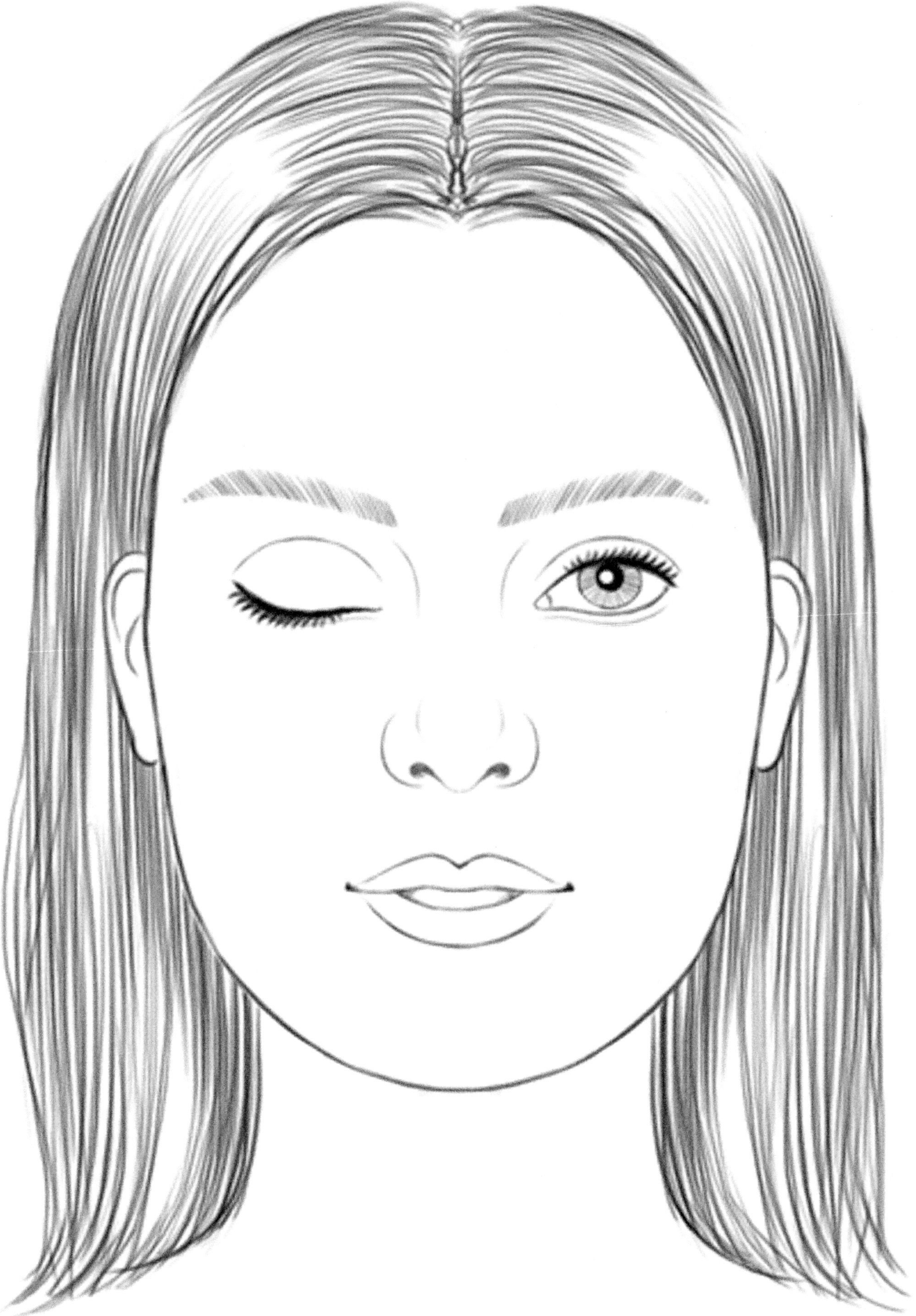

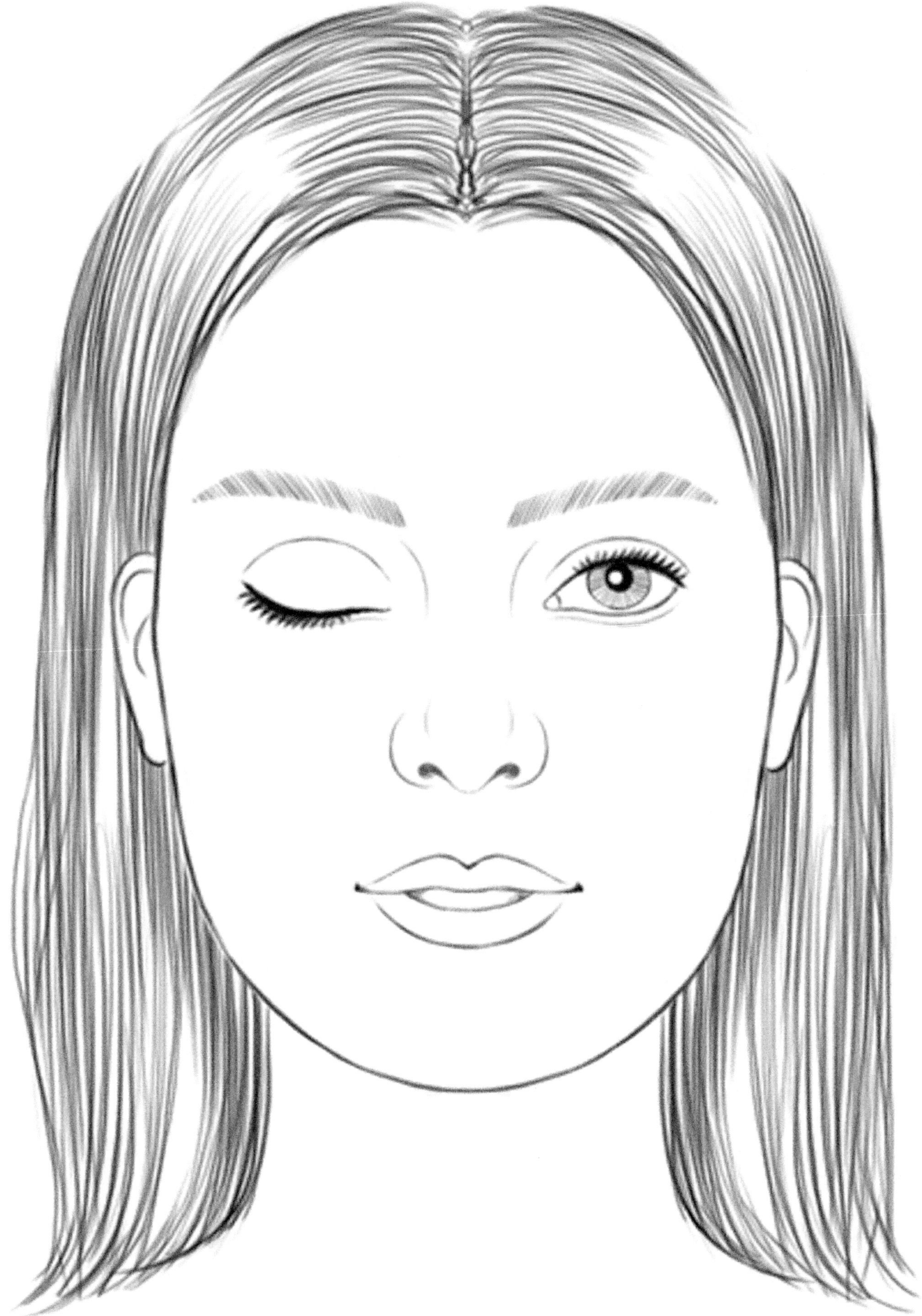

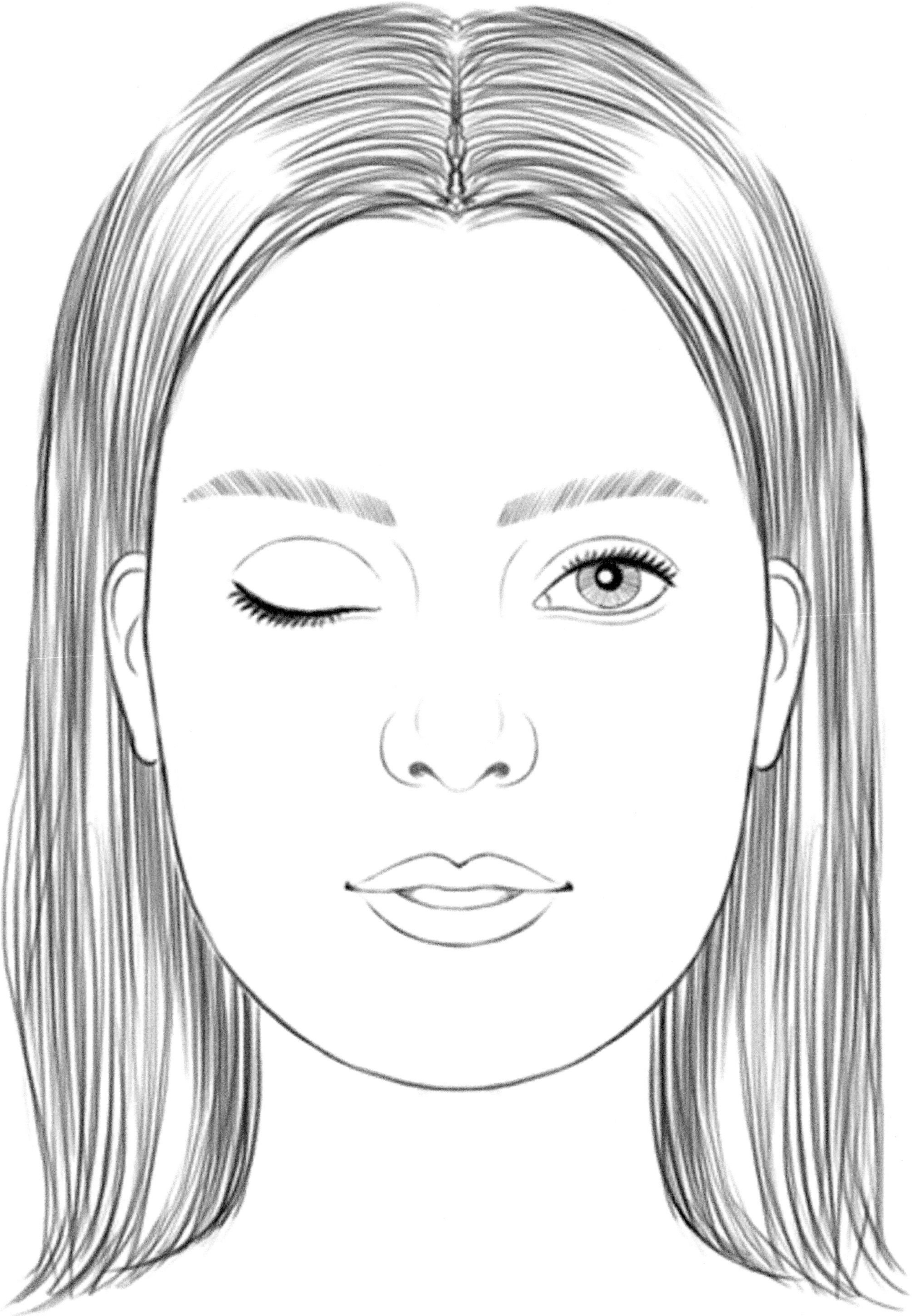

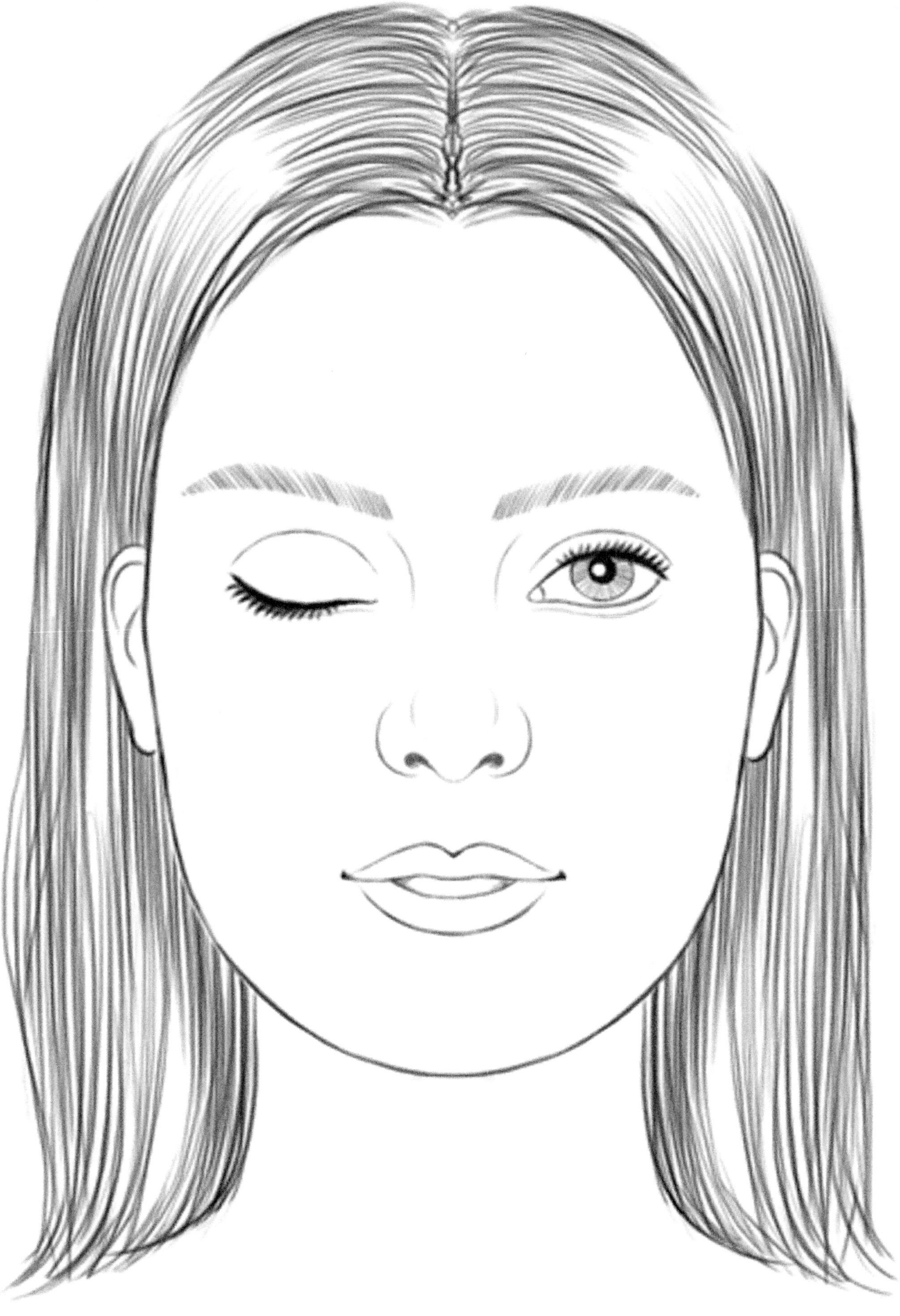

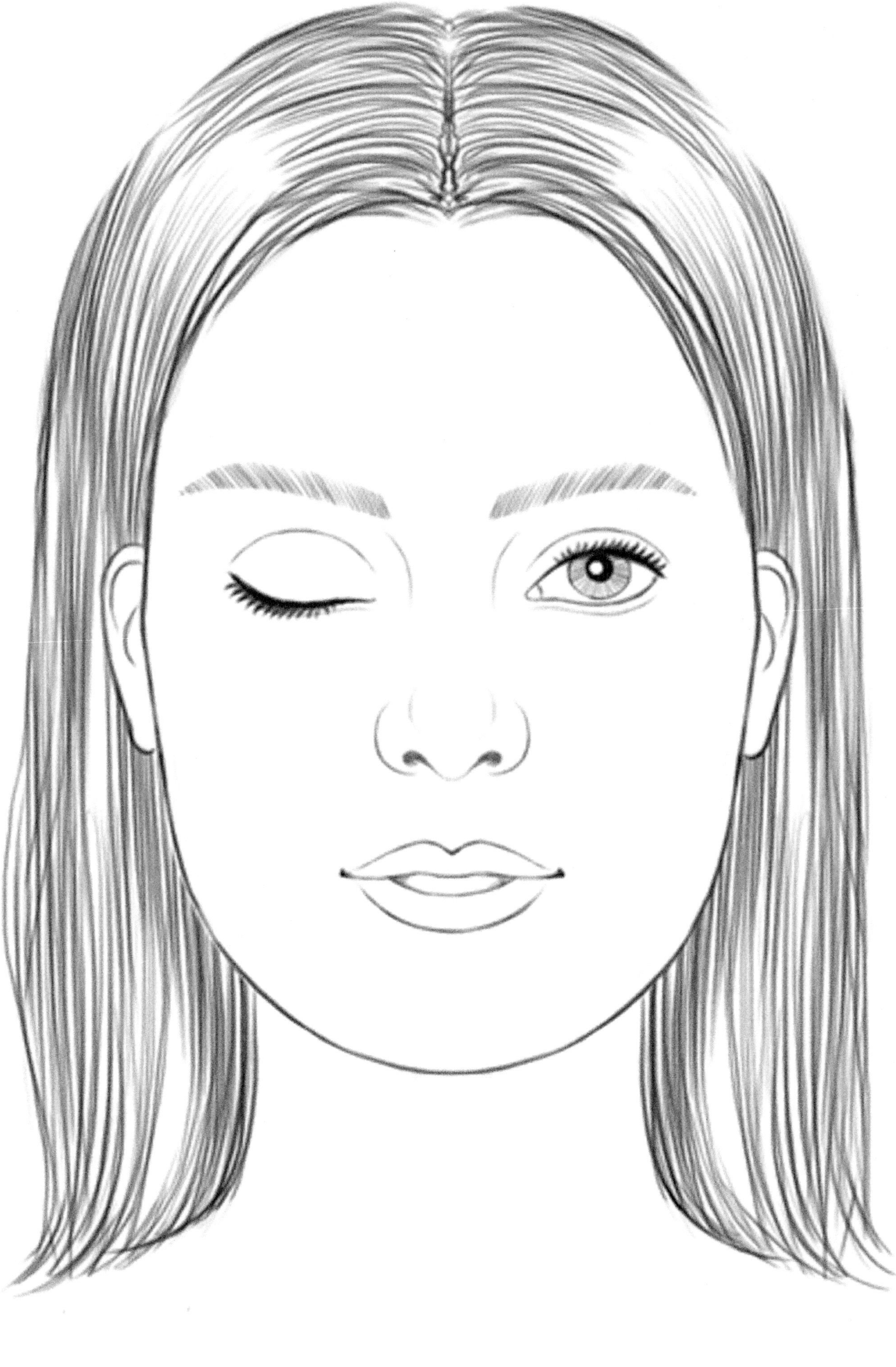

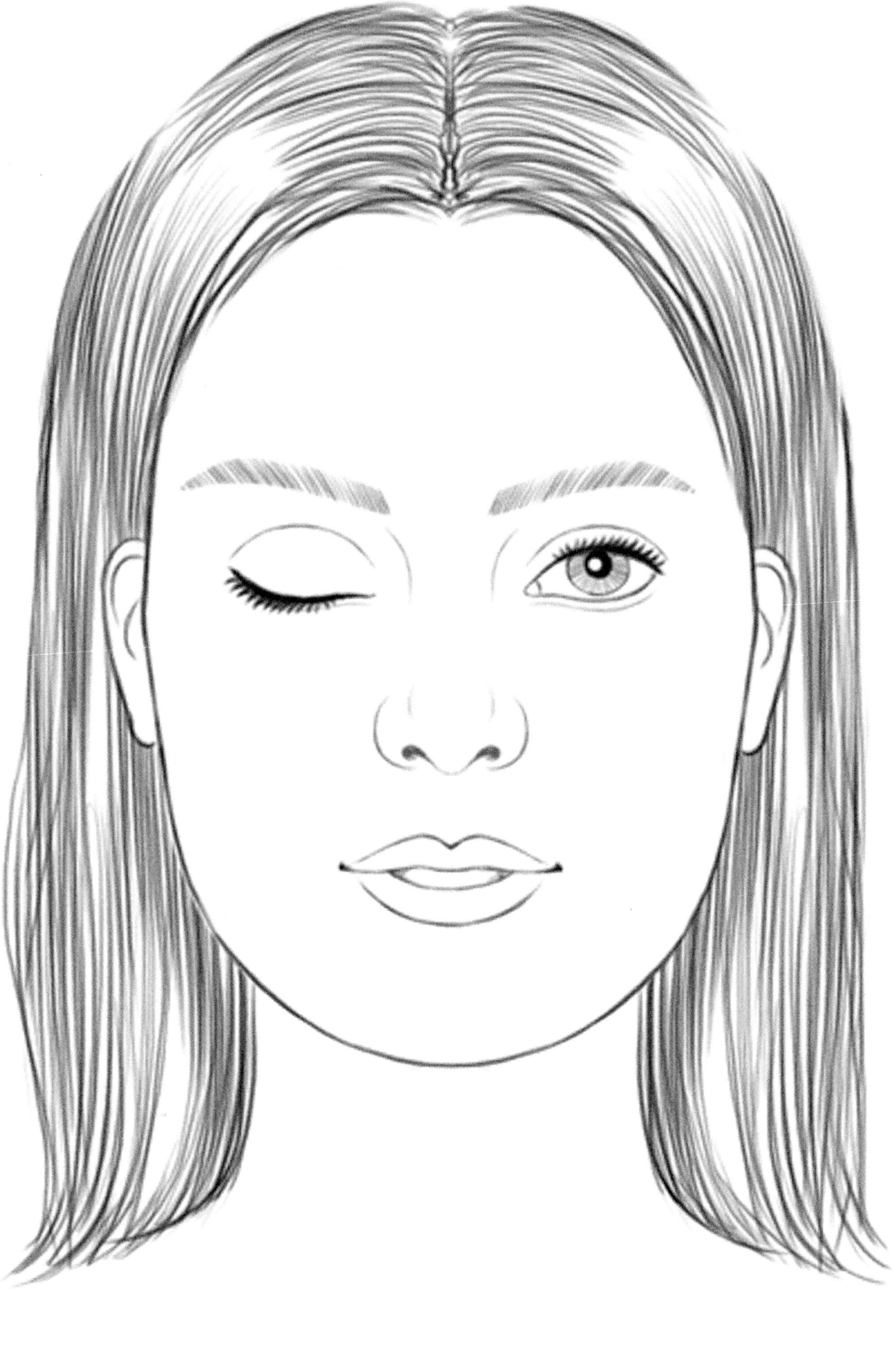

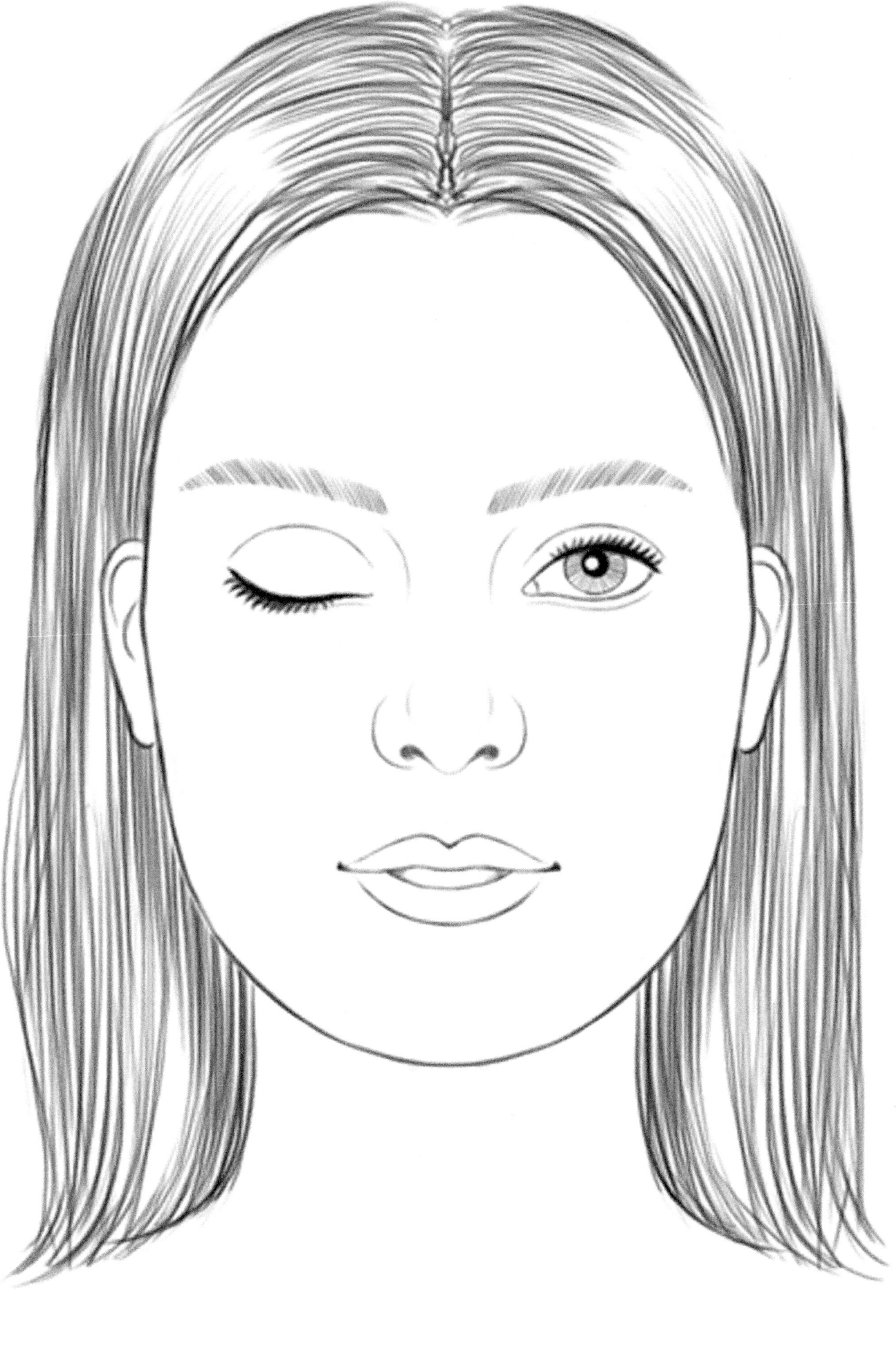

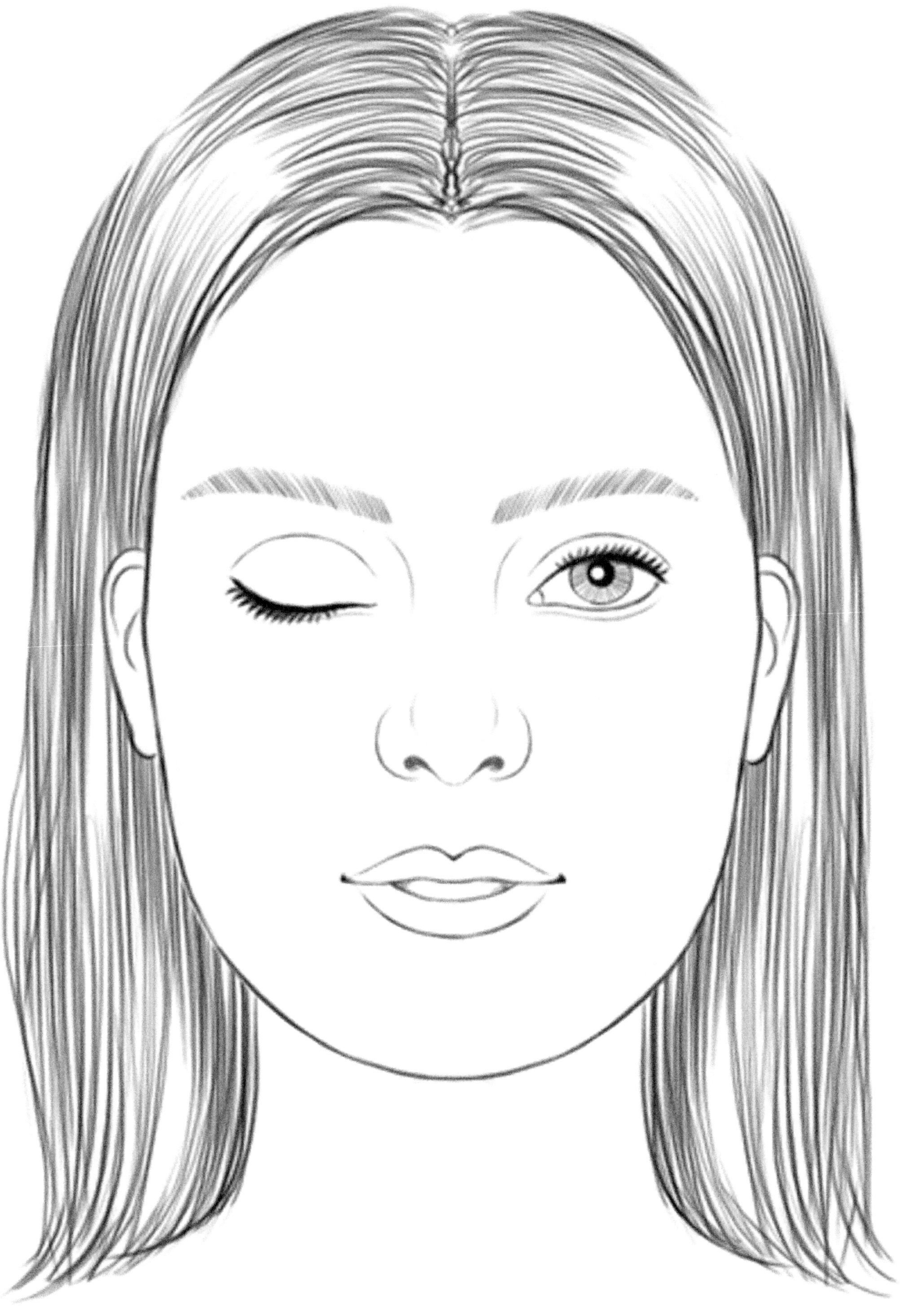

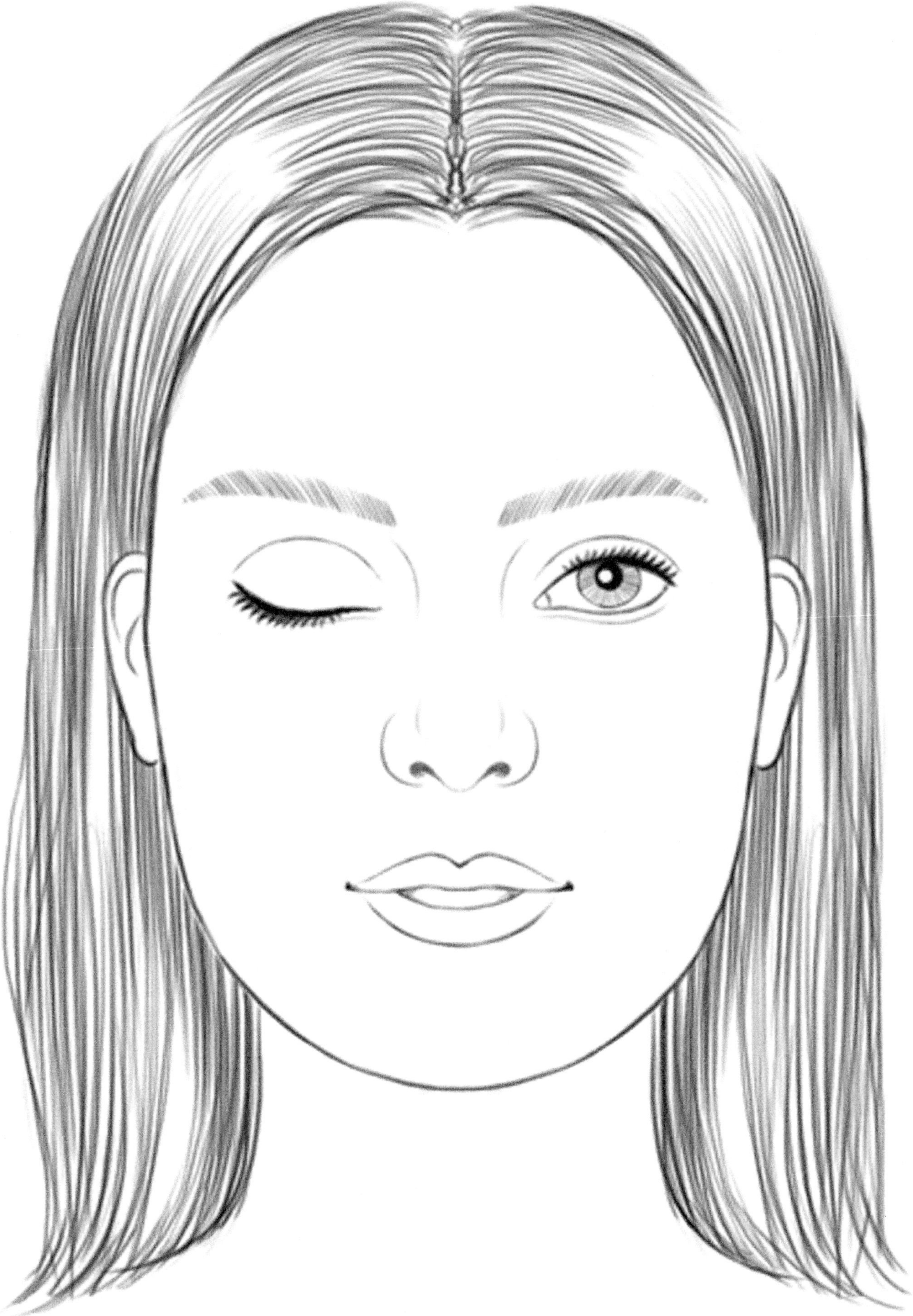

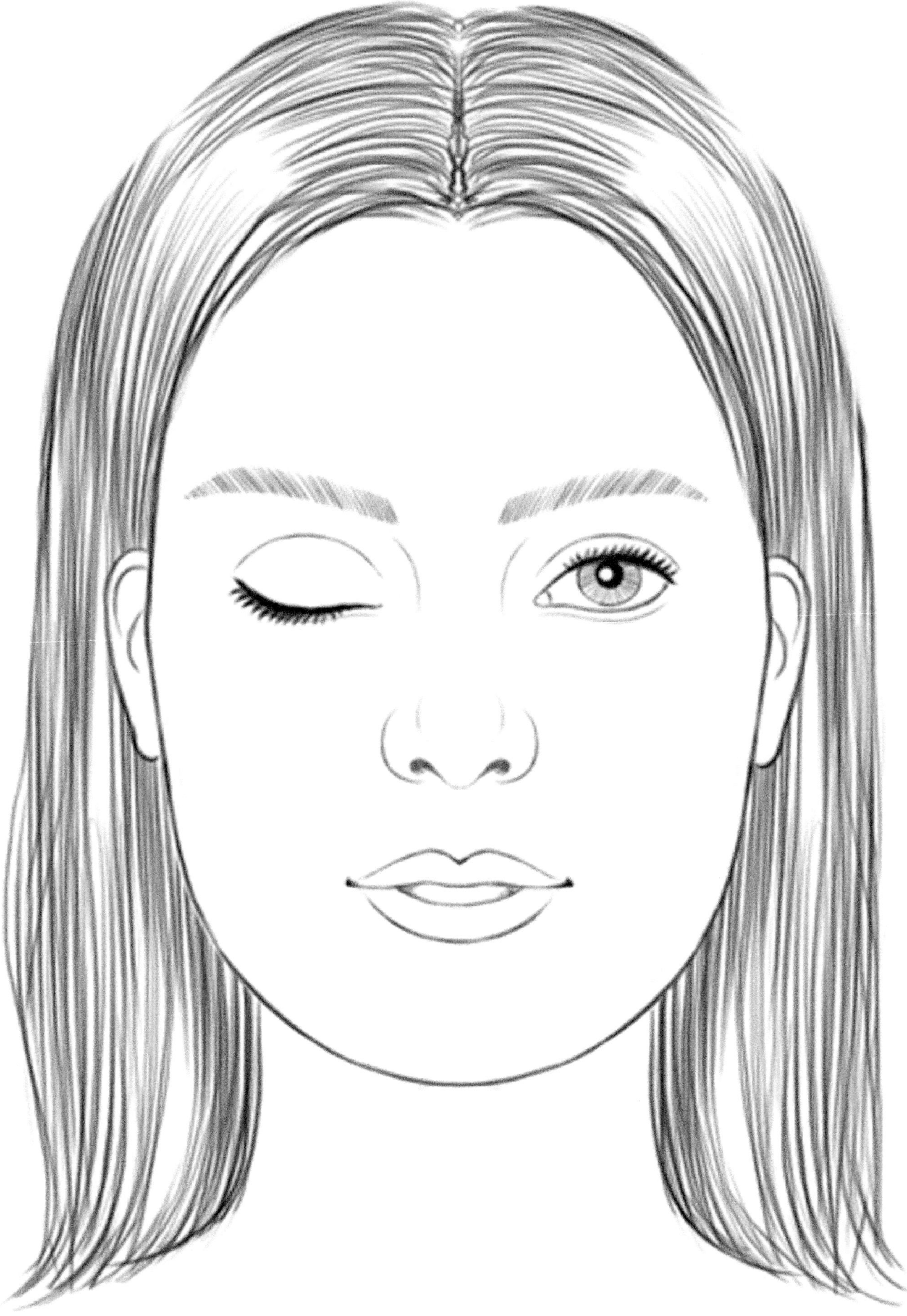

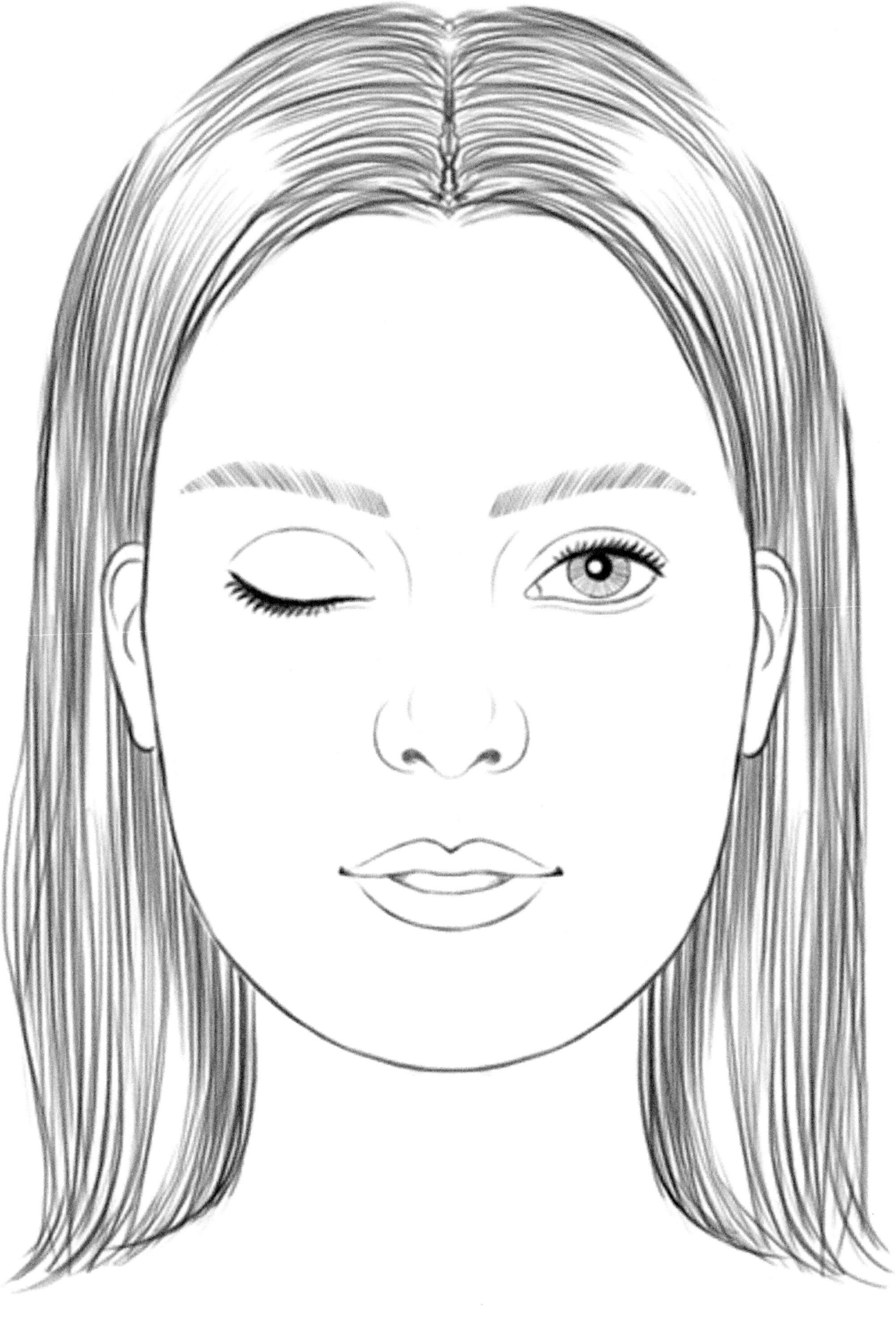

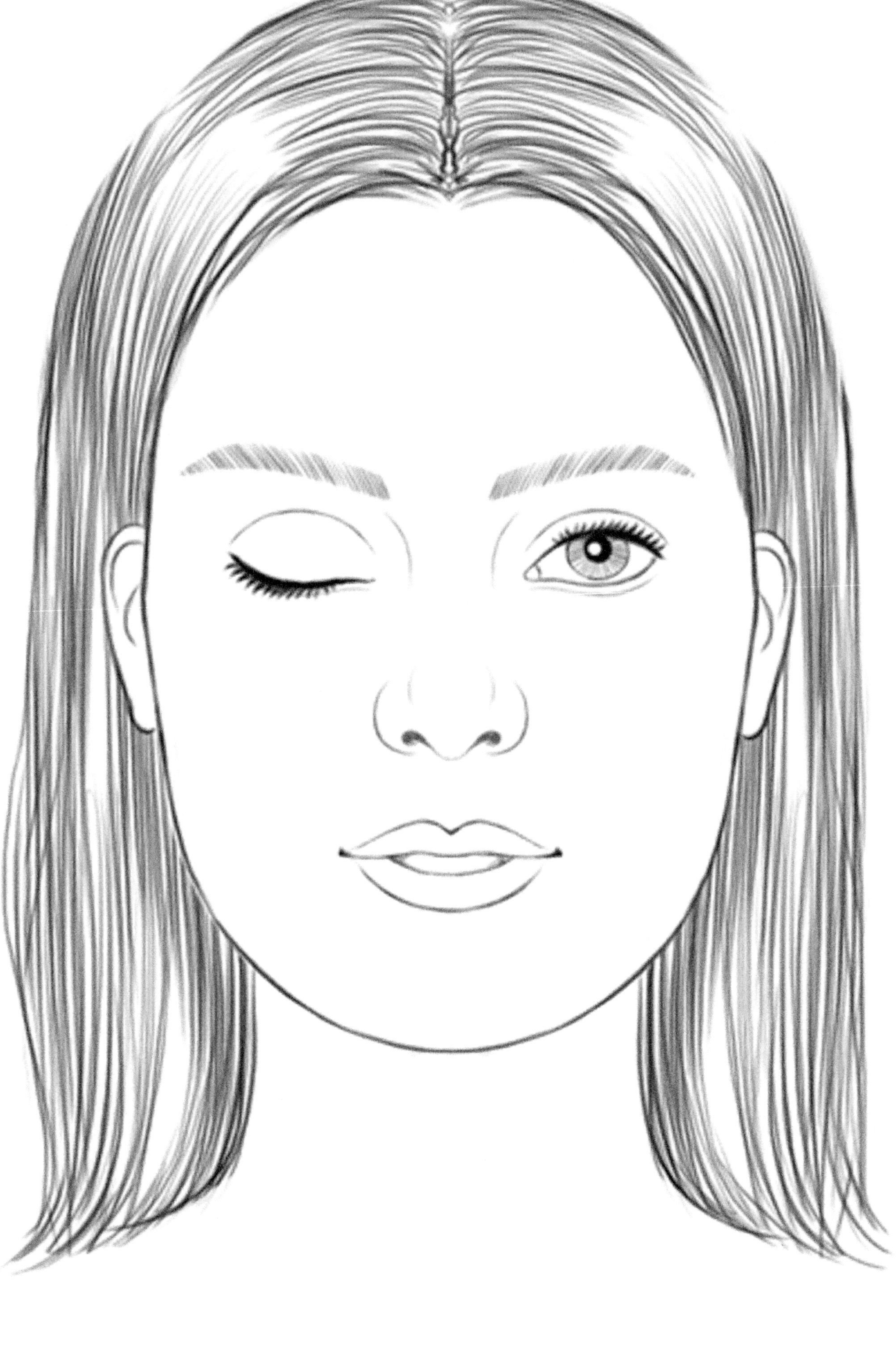

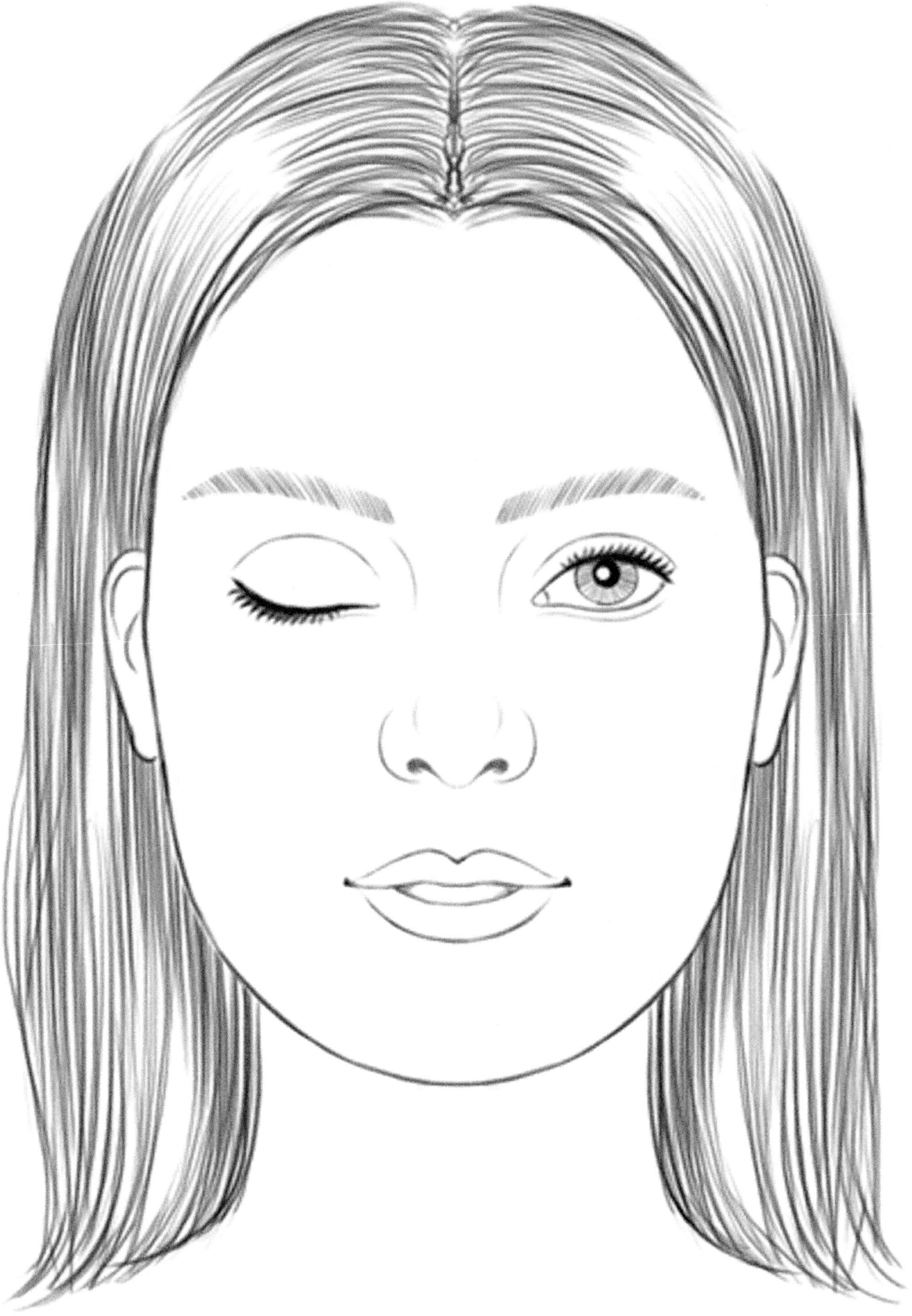

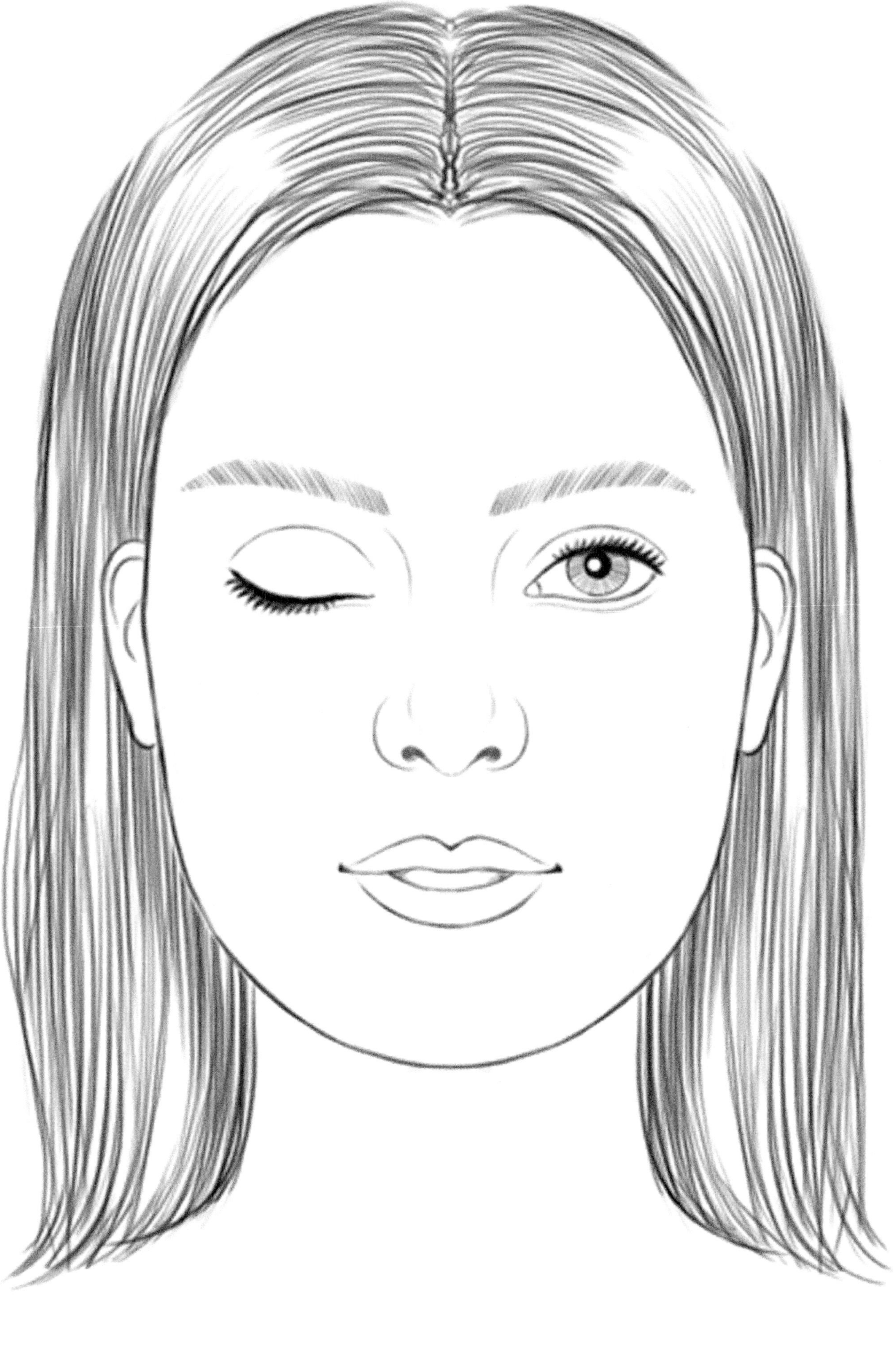

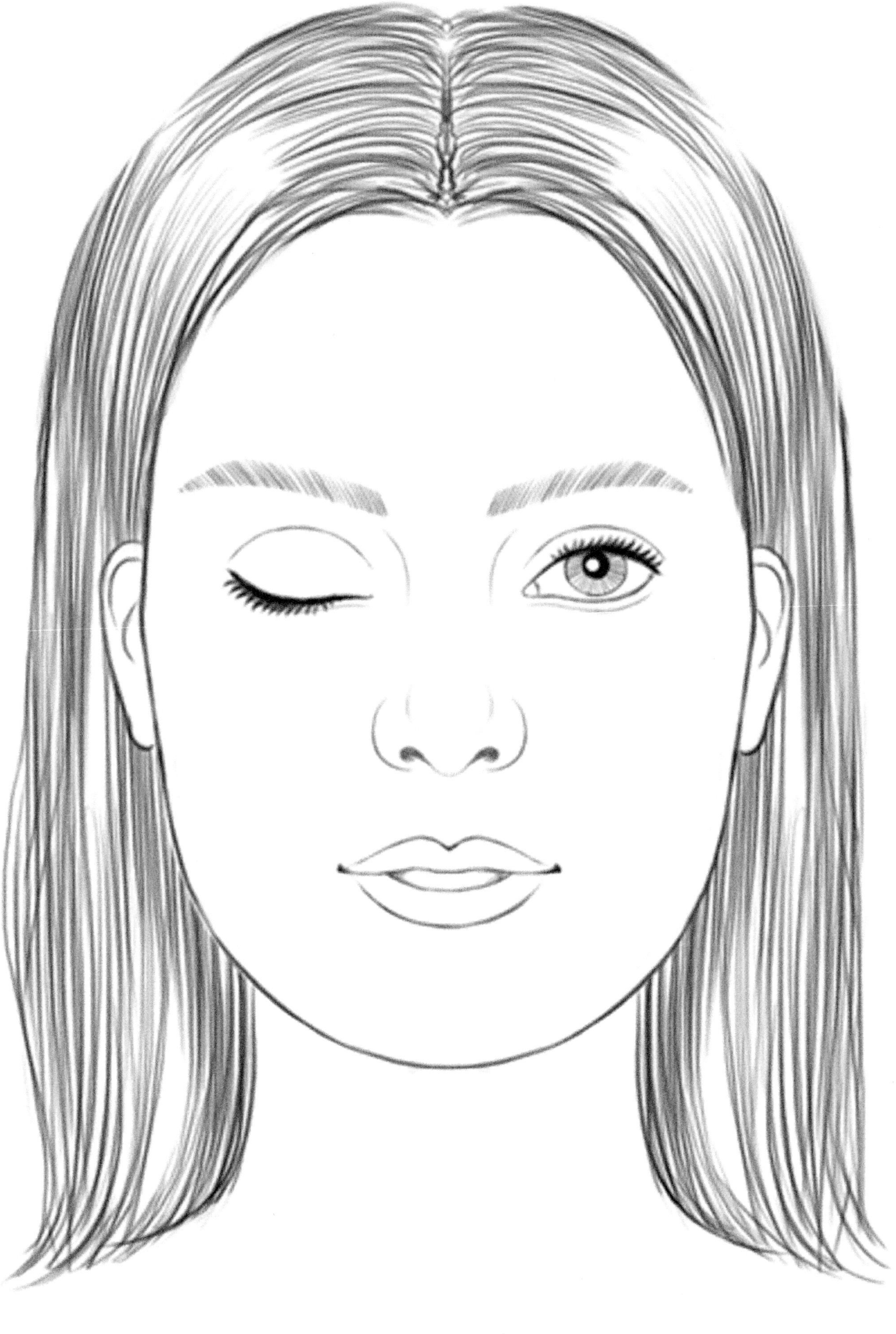

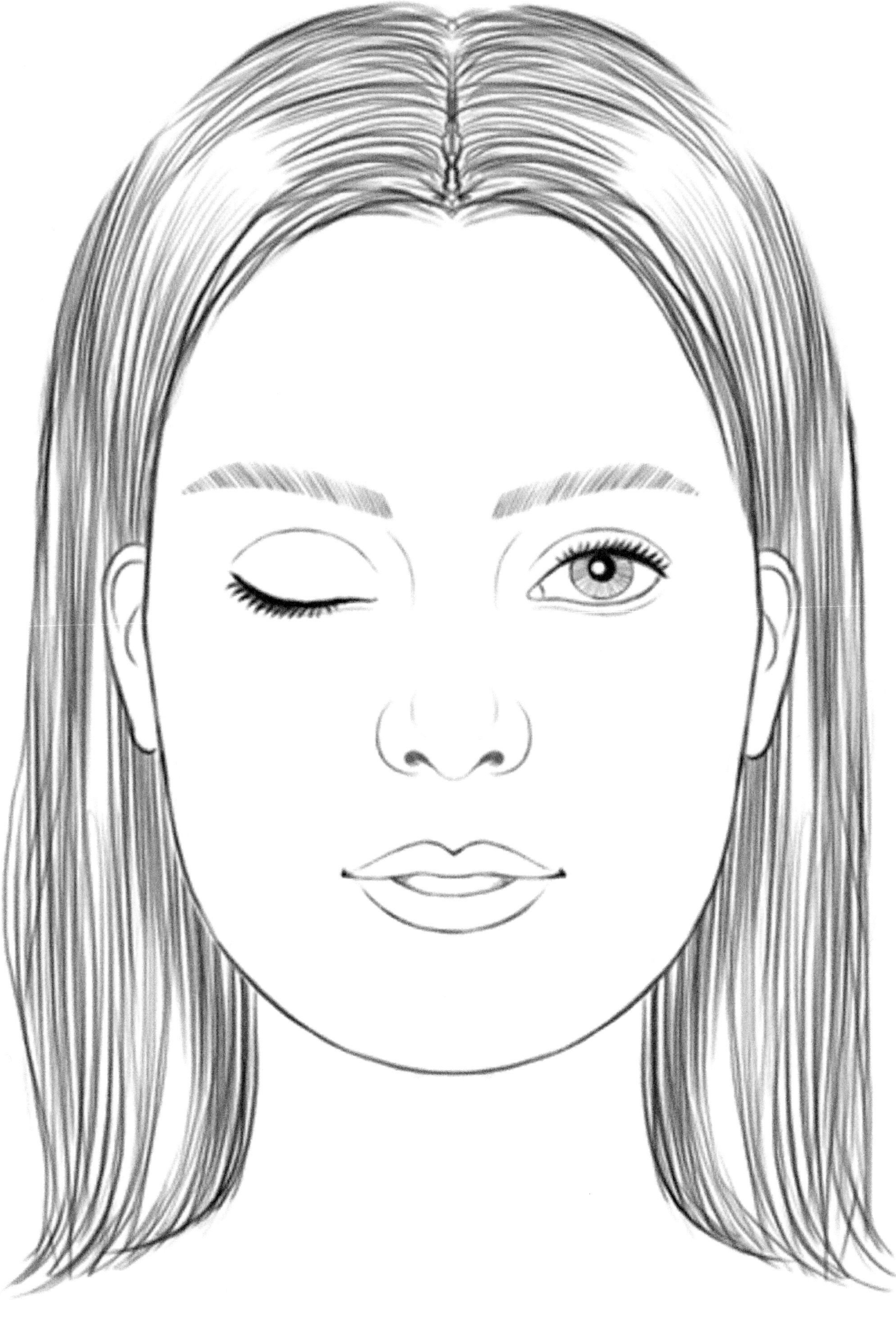

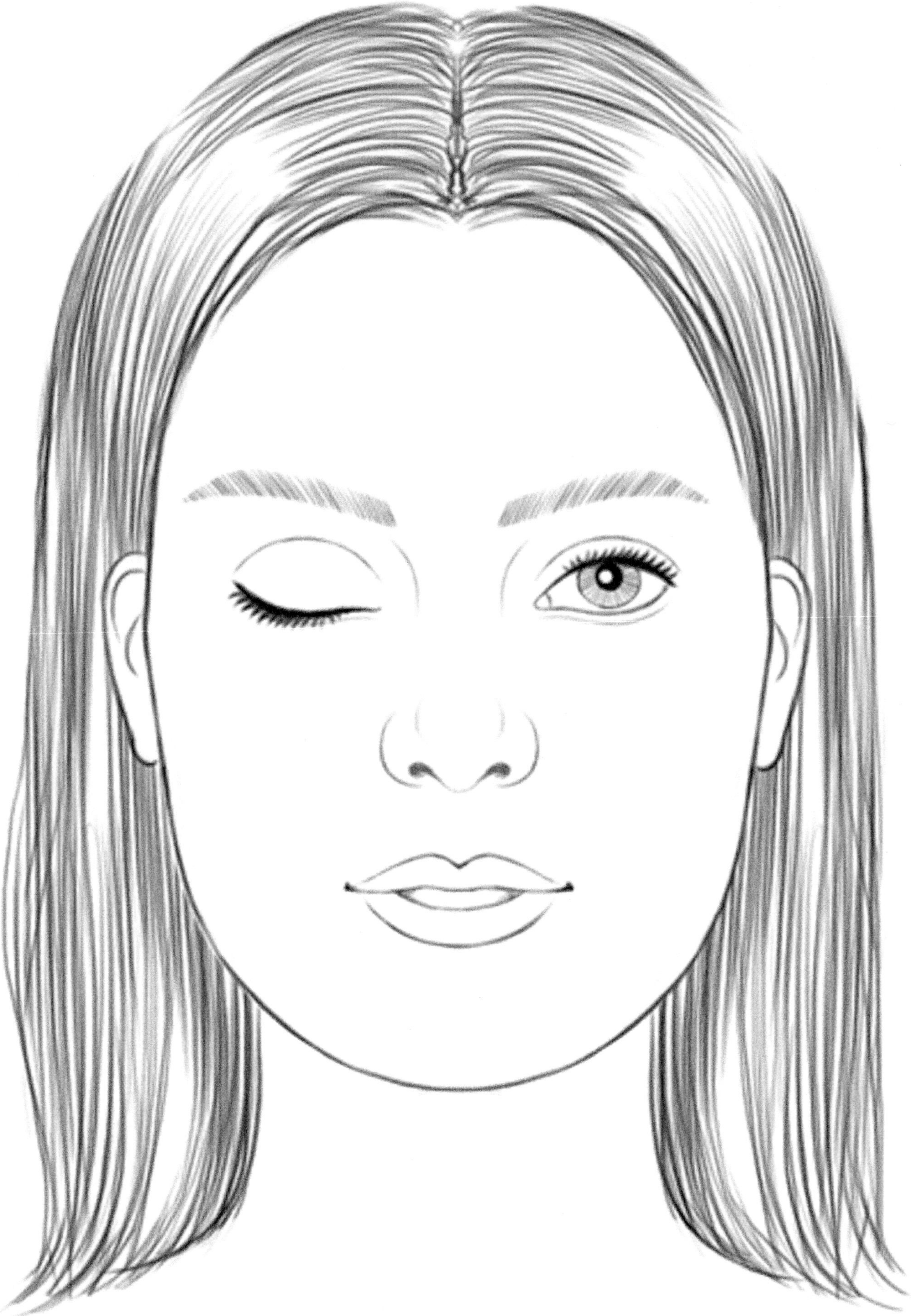

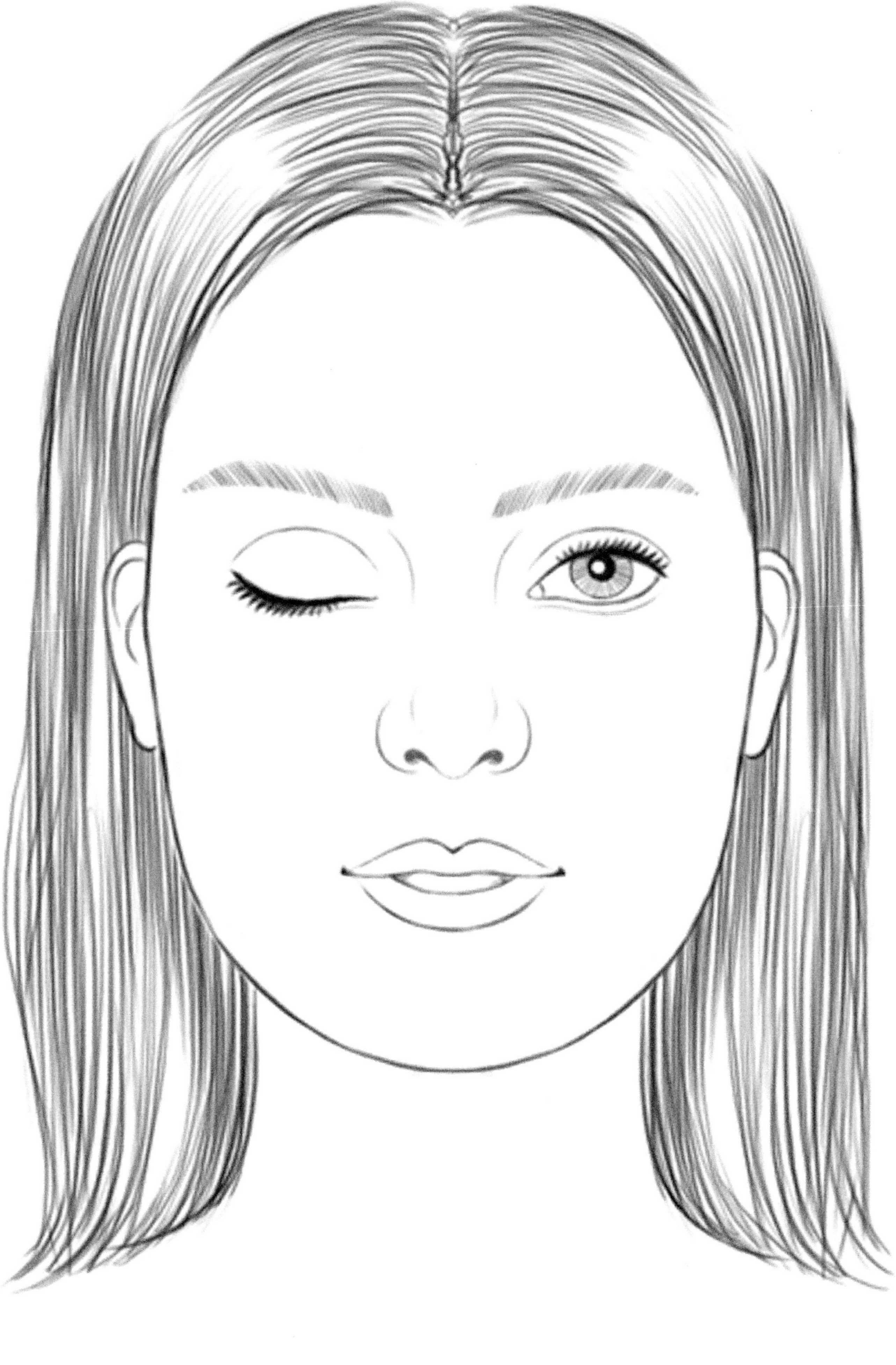

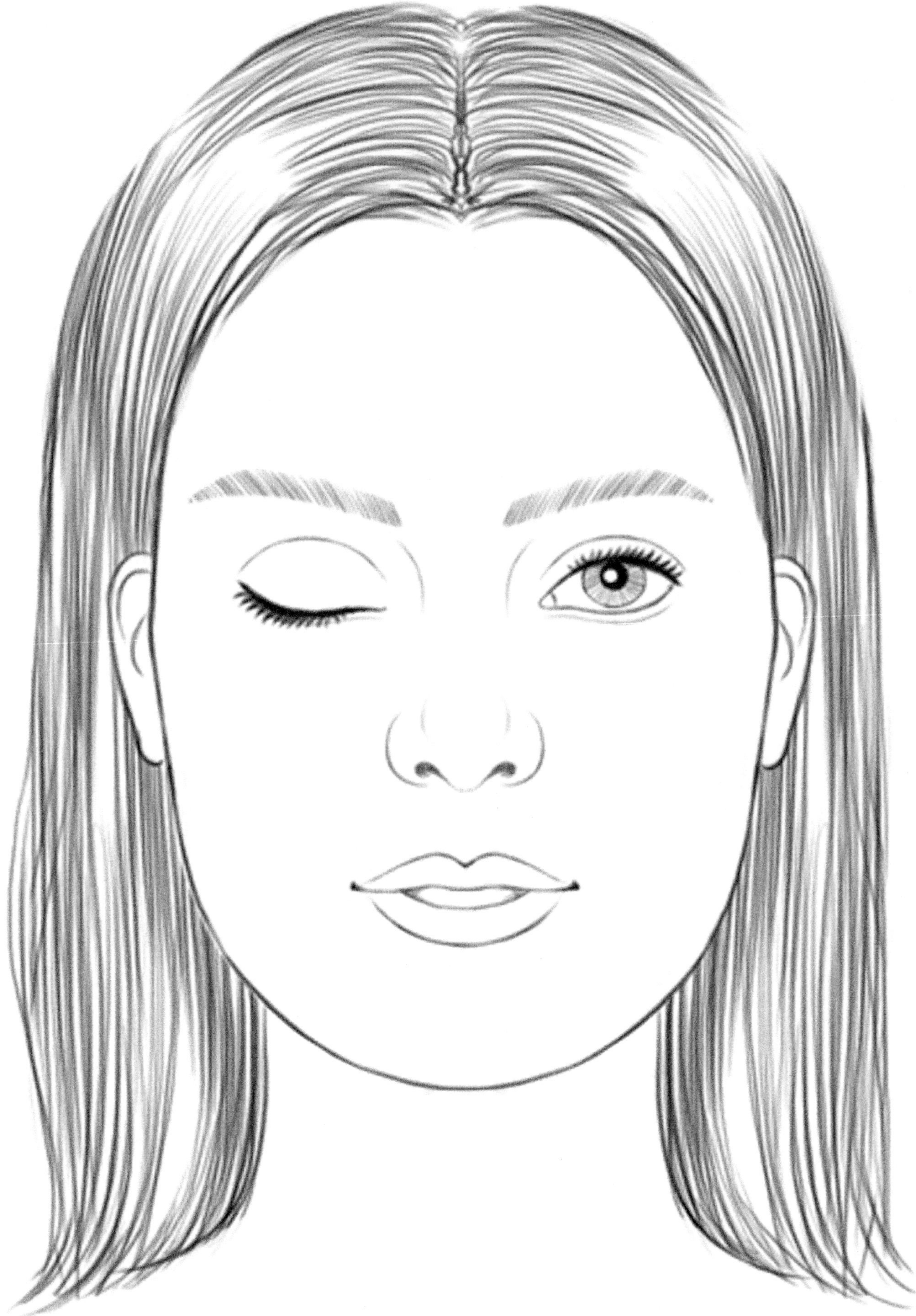

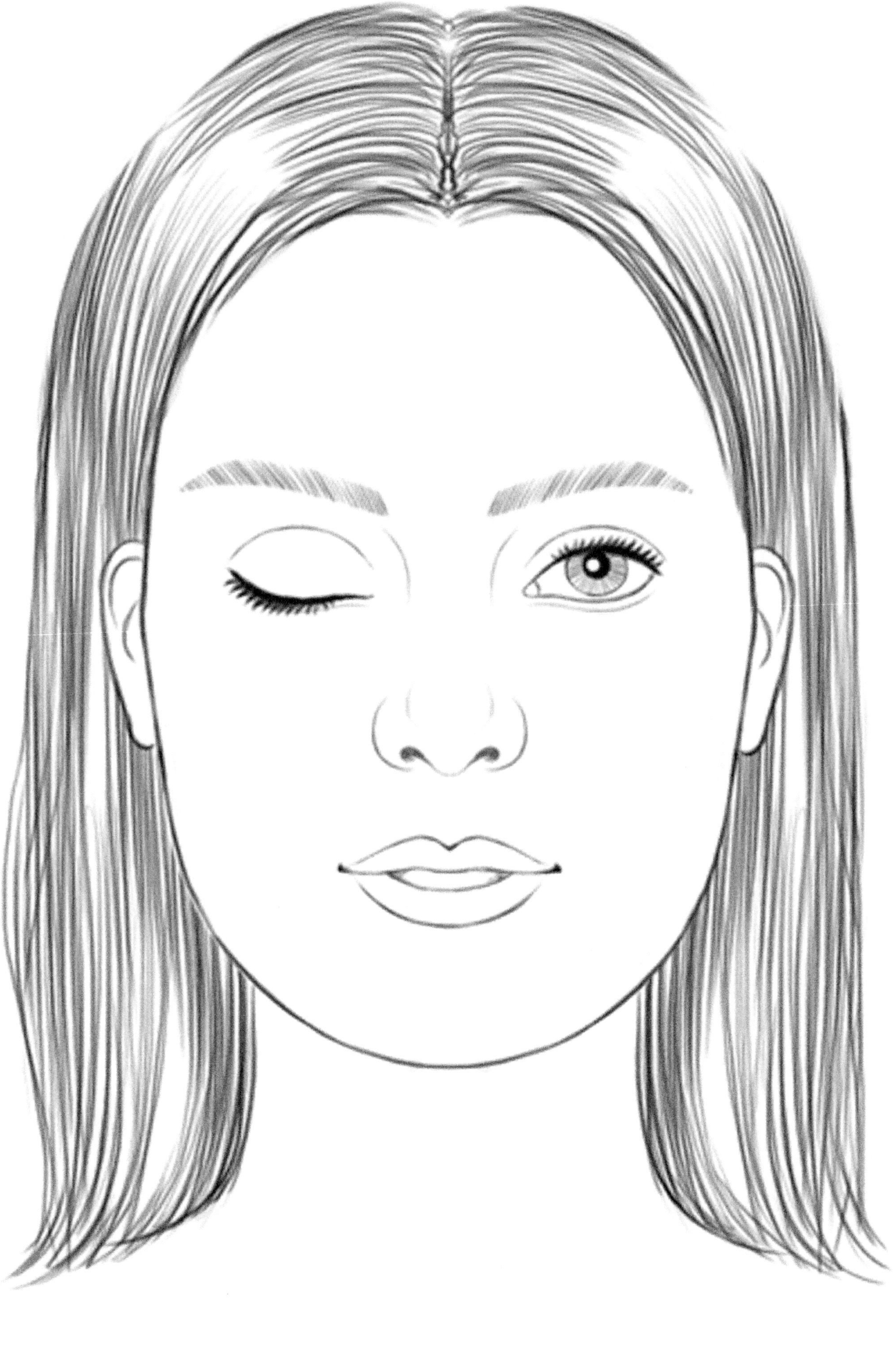

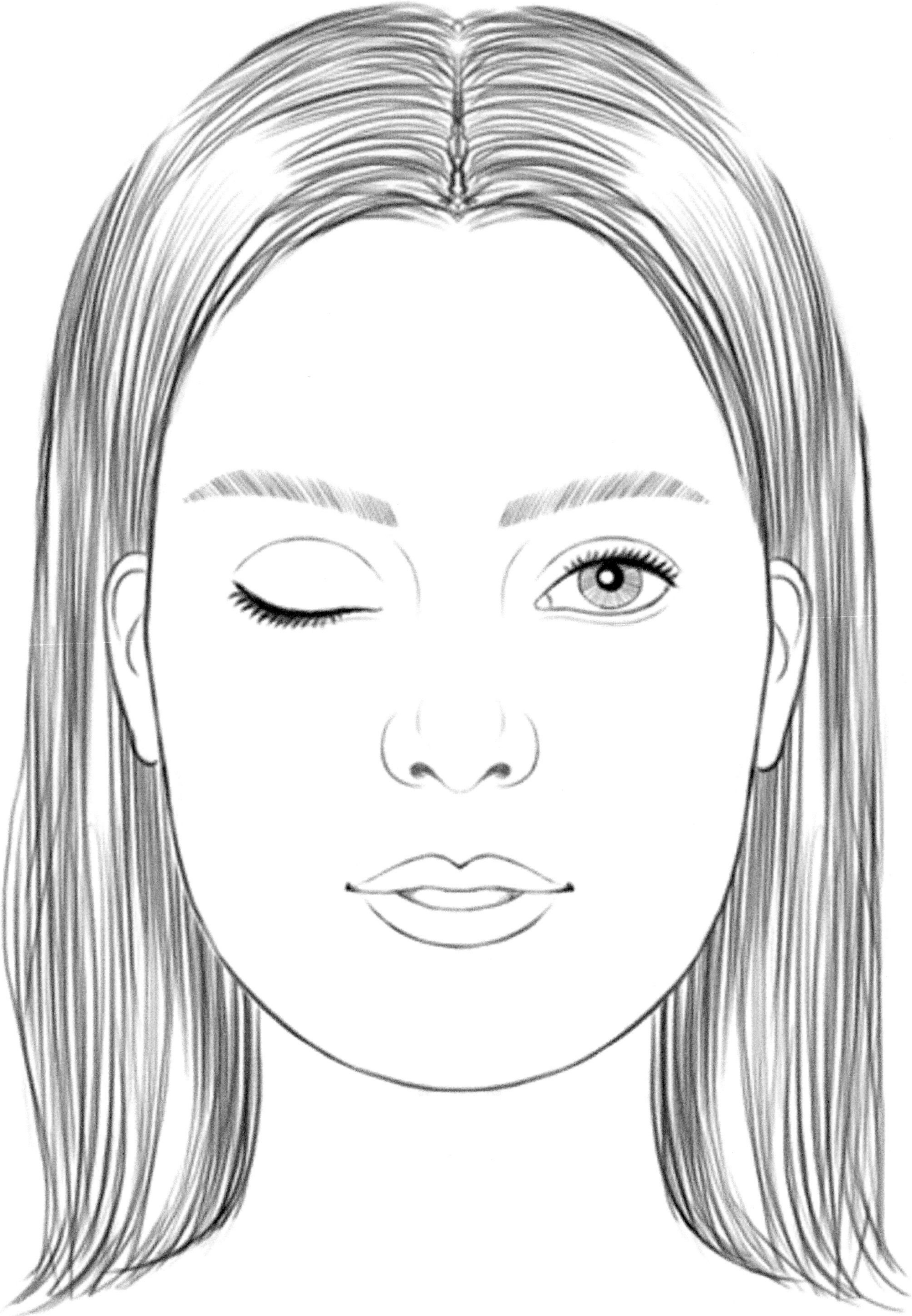

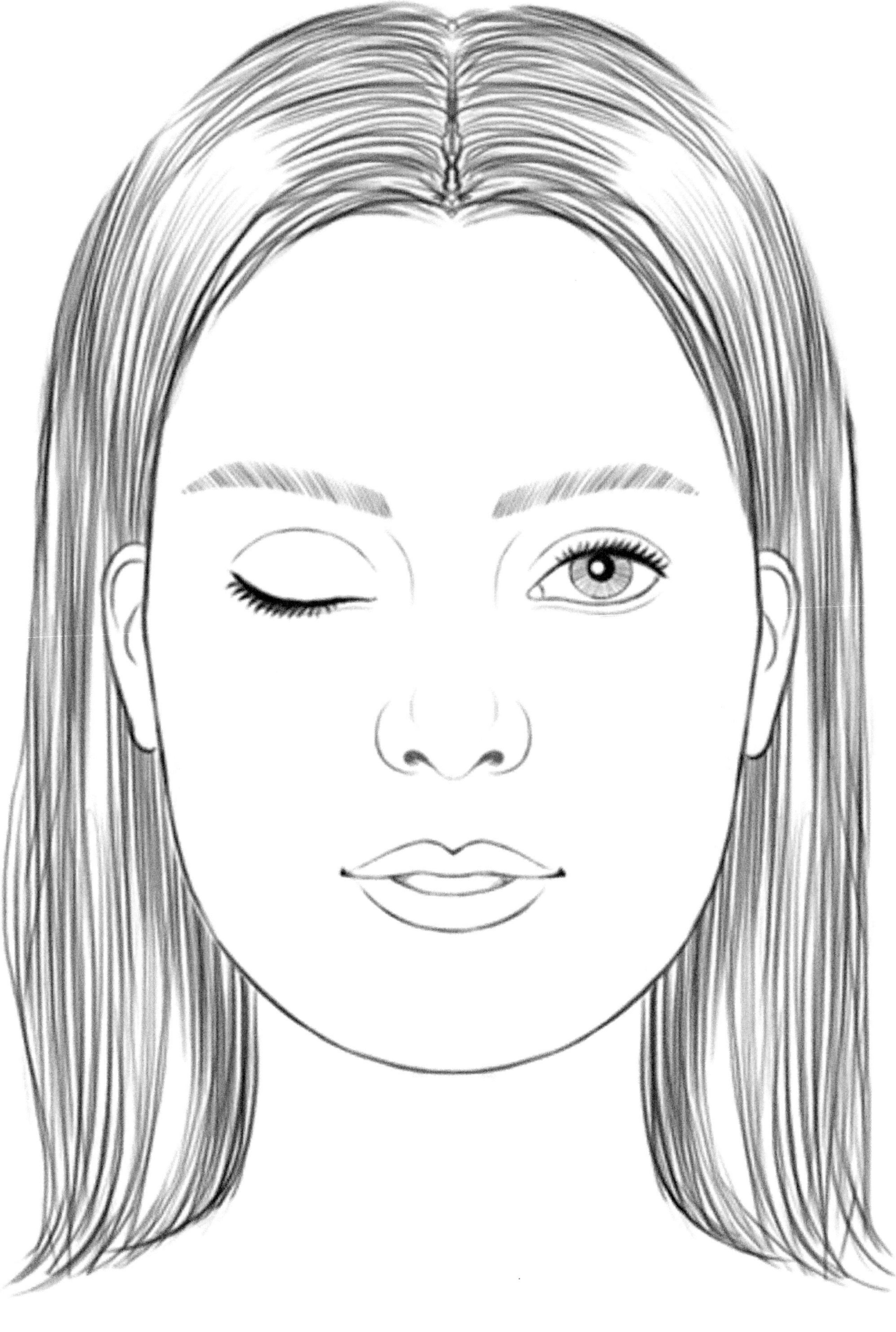

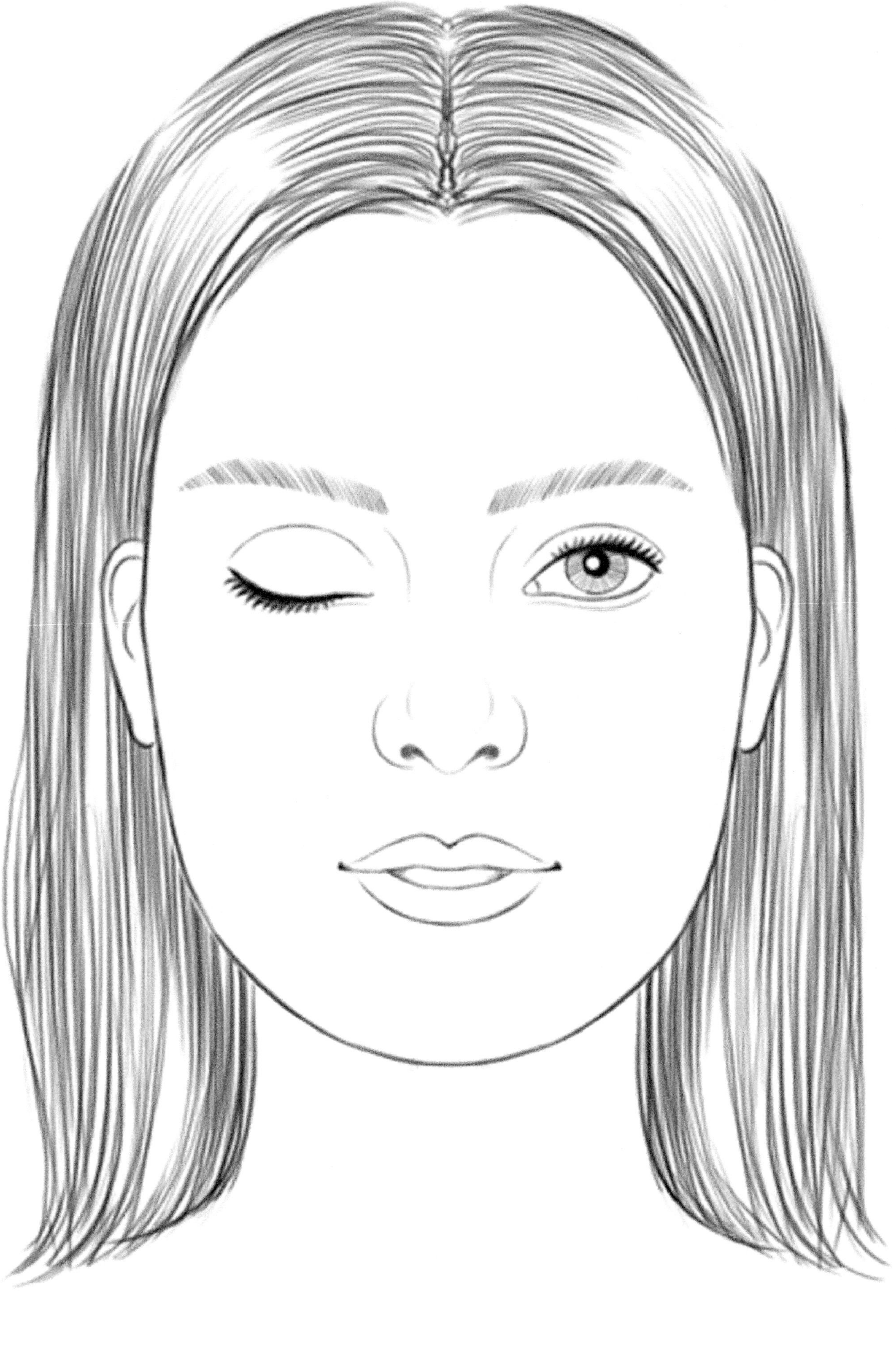

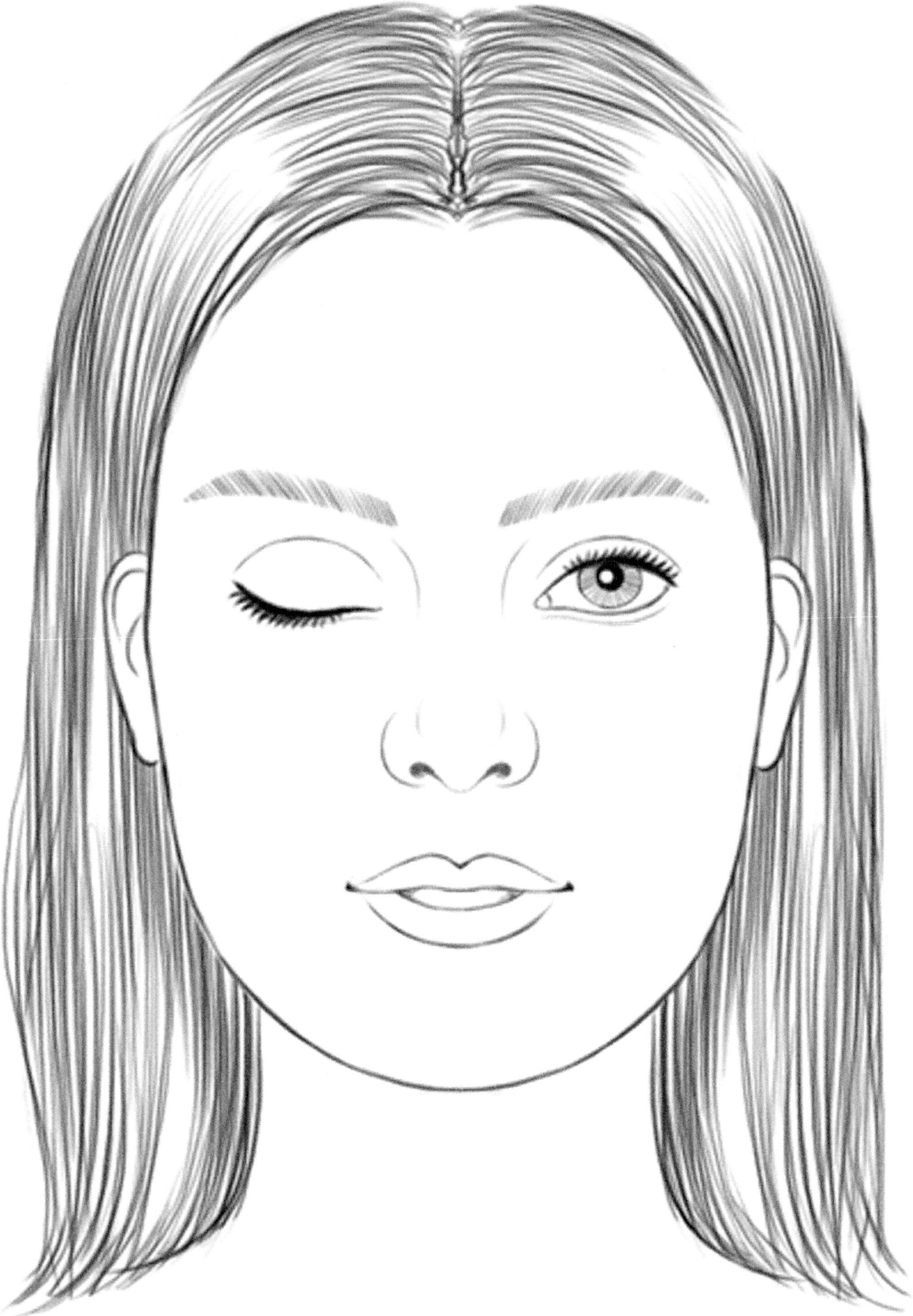

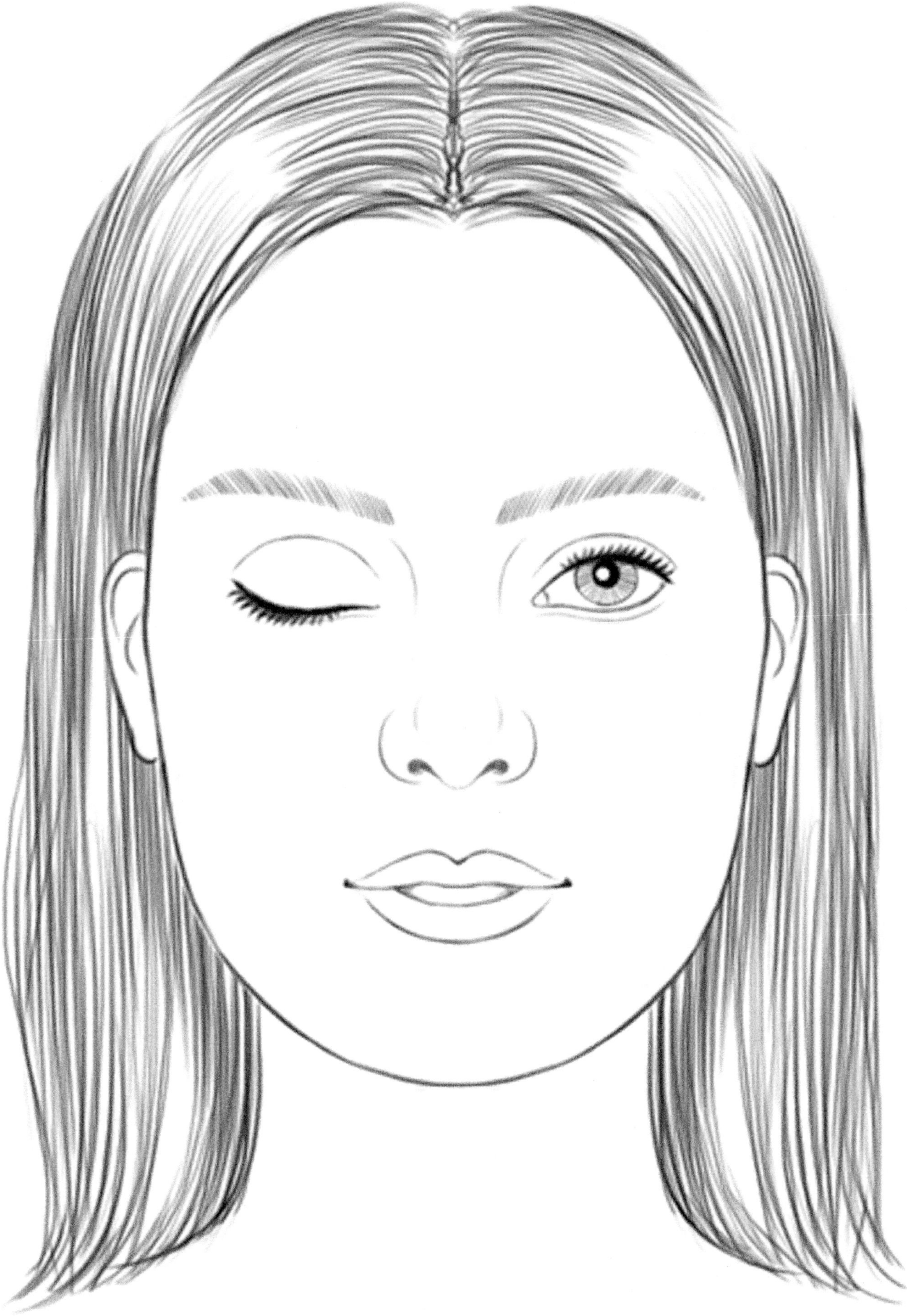

Printed in Great Britain
by Amazon

32808927R00059